psyche delicacies

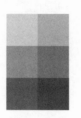

ALSO BY CHRIS KILHAM

Tales from the Medicine Trail
The Whole Food Bible
Kava: Medicine Hunting in Paradise
The Five Tibetans
In Search of the New Age
Take Charge of Your Health

psyche delicacies

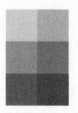

**coffee, chocolate, chiles,
kava, and cannabis, and
why they're good for you**

By Chris Kilham

RODALE

© 2001 by Chris Kilham

Cover photographs © by Dennie Cody/FPG International, Klaus Lahnstein/Stone

Printed in the United States of America

Rodale Inc. makes every effort to use acid-free ∞, recycled paper ♻.

Cover and Interior Designer: Christopher Rhoads
Photographers: Dennie Cody/FPG International, Klaus Lahnstein/Stone, Mitch Mandel/Rodale Images, Kurt Wilson/Rodale Images

Interior photographs courtesy of Chris Kilham

Library of Congress Cataloging-in-Publication Data

Kilham, Christopher.
  Psyche delicacies : coffee, chocolate, chiles, kava, and cannabis, and why they're good for you / By Chris Kilham.
    p.   cm.
  Includes index.
  ISBN 1–57954–347–2 hardcover
  1. Psychotropic plants—Health aspects.   I. Title.
RM315 .K53   2001
615'.788—dc21   2001004476

Distributed to the book trade by St. Martin's Press
2   4   6   8   10   9   7   5   3   1   hardcover

Visit us on the Web at www.rodalestore.com, or call us toll-free at (800) 848-4735.

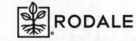

WE INSPIRE AND ENABLE PEOPLE TO IMPROVE
THEIR LIVES AND THE WORLD AROUND THEM

For Craig Weatherby, trusted friend and argonautic ally

(I know, it's your job)

Acknowledgments

I am grateful to many people for their support, assistance, and encouragement. Thanks to my wife, Shahannah Breedlove; my mother, Elizabeth Kilham; Lord Nelson, Ariipaea Salmon, Zachary and Hanna Gibson, K. C. Miller, and all my kind friends in Baie Martellie.

At Rodale, thanks to Nancy Hancock, Neil Wertheimer, Chris Potash, Jennifer Kushnier, Jim Gallucci, and all the other psyche delicacy–consuming baby boomers who championed this title and helped bring it to form.

Thanks to all my friends, associates, and tribal allies whose love, kindness, consideration, hospitality, support, humor, and humanity give me strength and inspiration and keep me going. Blessings to you all.

Viva la revolution!

Contents

Chiles—Hellfire in Your Mouth   86

Kava—The Pacific Elixir   122

Cannabis—Ganja Road   161

Introduction
The "Higher" Plants

The human fascination with and craving for mind-altering and mood-modifying plants stretches far back into history. Early archaeological excavations show that our primitive forebears were enamored of the opium poppy and cannabis along with other psychoactive seeds, barks, and flowers. The history of virtually every culture save those living at the icy poles gives testimony to the enduring human affinity for psychoactivity.

Psyche Delicacies explores the history, legends, lore, and reported uses of five extremely popular psychoactive plants—coffee, chocolate, chiles, kava (also known as kava kava), and cannabis (also known as marijuana, pot, ganja, grass, weed, reefer, dope, hemp, bhang, dagga, tea, boo, mary jane, muggles, charas, goddess, viper, pakololo, hay, kif, and smoke, to name just a few)—showing that in each case, the plant in question imparts benefits to both body and mind with little risk to health when used responsibly. These benefits explain why these five are among the most widely consumed and traded plants in the world. People by the hundreds of millions have embraced their use, spreading them from one country to another while inventing a multitude of ingenious ways to consume them.

According to strict botanical terminology, the "higher plants" are those flora that possess well-developed physical characteristics such as flowers and fruits. By this description, apple trees, roses, vanilla vines, and squash plants all qualify as higher plants. I have other criteria. For the purposes of this book, I propose that the "higher" plants are those flora that make themselves uniquely valuable to humans by virtue of the desirable influence they exert upon our minds. As a result of their mood-modifying allure, we are so enamored of these plants that we cultivate them anywhere and everywhere they will grow. We become their advocates, their porters, their protectors, their proclaimers. You could say, even, that they have us under a spell.

We derive pleasure from plants through all our senses. Many flowers are so lovely in color and form as to delight the eye and provoke the mind with their beauty. The sound of leaves rustling in a breeze stirs the imagination, conjuring the sensation of a natural symphony. Succulent fruits so tease the taste buds as to be spoken of in the most provocative and sensual of terms. Aromas released from blossoms, grasses, barks, and other plant parts tickle the olfactory bulb and tantalize our reptilian brains. The feeling of touching, being brushed by, or lying in vegetation engenders a pleasurable sense of connectedness with the natural world, with which we are inextricably intertwined.

So too, certain plants when ingested produce feelings, sensations, and an overall condition of body and mind that we want to experience over and over again. Coffee, chocolate, chiles, kava, and cannabis are akin in that they modify both mind and mood and their use is sought after by aficionados worldwide. In each case, these plants have been praised and excoriated, promoted and banned, embraced and spurned for their salutary effects. Across history and time, pleasure seekers

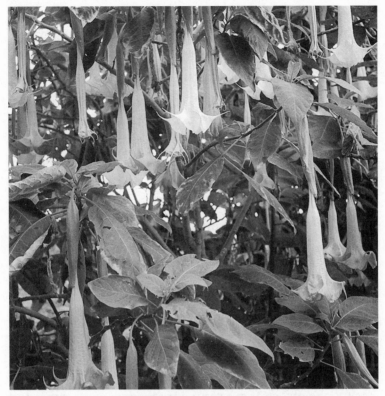

Brugmansia, a beautiful and potent shamanic hallucinogen, is most definitely a "higher" plant.

and pleasure haters have fought acrimonious battles over these user-friendly, healthful plants, these delightful psyche delicacies.

Language shapes our way of thinking about things, and the language of psychoactive substances is heavily loaded with cognitive cultural baggage. Thus I choose most often to employ the term *reverie* to describe the psychosomatic effects produced by the five psyche delicacies at hand, using terms like *high* and *stoned* more sparingly. Typically referring to daydreaming or being lost in thought, *reverie* implies a reflective condition of mind that is consistent with the use of the psyche delicacies.

Once humans became smitten with the reverie that these "higher" plants give rise to, their broad distribution was all but guaranteed. It is a brilliant Darwinian evolutionary scheme. Plants secrete chemical compounds to ward off invasion by bacteria, fungi, and predators. They muster natural defenses against exposure to extreme degrees of wind, sun, heat, and cold. They mimic the sexual pheromones of certain insects to ensure that they will be pollinated by members of those particular species. And they create psychoactive compounds that so delight the human mind as to ensure their broad distribution. Plants are far more resourceful than most people are willing to believe. They have learned how to influence our minds, and they do so brilliantly.

In every case, the plants featured in *Psyche Delicacies* once existed in relative obscurity. But as quickly as they were discovered, they spread like wildfire from one nation to another, even leaping across oceans. Each plant has undergone a long and extraordinary journey and continues to do so to this day. Each is the object of substantial trade; each is the subject of scientific and medical scrutiny; and each produces its own precious reverie.

So why focus on just these five plants and not others? First of all, they are by far the most commonly used psychoactives in the world. Then, the psyche delicacies featured in this book occupy a special place within the range of plants that affect the mind. St. John's wort and ginkgo, for example, act upon the brain as well, but they do not inspire reverie. Tobacco and grain-based alcoholic beverages unquestionably alter mind and mood, but both are associated with grave risks to health. And plant-based agents such as peyote, hallucinogenic mushrooms, and other like substances are so potent in their effects that one cannot take them and still carry on with the activities of daily life. (I have a high regard for those agents, for they are valuable sacred tools, but they are not appropriate for regular, everyday use.) By contrast, coffee, chocolate, chiles, kava, and cannabis can fit well into a healthy, active lifestyle with little or no harmful effects.

The plants found here in *Psyche Delicacies* are exquisite works of nature arising from the murky, protoplasmic swamp of biological history. We may never know the full story of how these plants came into being or exactly how they came by their special gifts, but we do know with certainty that since their discovery and rediscovery by various cultures, they have swept over humankind like a great tidal surge. And just as we have carried these plants far and wide, so too have they borne the human mind on clouds of wonder. Thus, they are to us as gifts from the gods.

psyche
delicacies

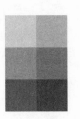

Coffee
The Noble Bean

My day begins with coffee, unless I am someplace where it is made so poorly that drinking it is a heinous assault upon the senses, or if it is, for whatever reason, completely unavailable. Thankfully, those days are rare. Usually I am up in the fives; my wife, Shahannah, does not budge. After a bracing shower, I descend to the kitchen—my coffee laboratory.

Preparing the morning's coffee is a task I approach with meticulous care and devotion. I have, by fastidious trial and error, figured the exact measure of whole beans to brew a large thermos of the stuff: dark, rich, and fragrant. I prefer the big bold Indonesian or African varieties, like Sumatra or Kenya AA. Even better if the coffee is organically grown, without toxic agricultural chemicals. The grinding is loud, but still my wife does not stir. I patiently place the fine grind into a paper filter—unbleached of course, no dioxin—and pour with exacting care the freshly boiled spring water. The pouring process must be accomplished such that the water comes in contact with all the grounds evenly, ensuring the strongest brew. If you bring Zenlike precision to the making of coffee, it will deliver bliss: Practice yields perfection, and perfection is worth the practice.

Only when the coffee is made and I am ensured of a fragrant and lively brew that will embolden the spirit, rally the mind like a clarion call, and open the eyes wide to the clear beaming light of day, do I then stand at the foot of the stairs and call to Shahannah. Sometimes I carry a cup upstairs and slip the rim of it under her nose, allowing the nutty, aromatic vapors to woo her forth from the boggy peat of sleep. As her nostrils flare, her heavy lids open, and voilà! It's a wonderful new day. The perfect cup of coffee wipes clean the windows of perception to sparkling, glassy brilliance.

Heaven in a Cup

I am convinced that Hell is not as Dante depicted, all fire and torment and helpless souls chained to walls, flesh being pulled off in chunks without end, Amen. No, Hell is a place of eternal dullness devoid of sense or sensation, a joyless realm of complete indifference. There, the coffee is execrable. Harsh beans, poorly roasted, are ground too coarse and used sparingly, producing a thin brown water that burns for hours on a Bunn-O-Matic until the vapors smell like a soiled scrub sponge that has been kept damp in a dark sink cabinet. In Hell there is no reverie.

But in Boston, the city where I was born and outside of which I now reside, it's a different story. For years, the very best cup of coffee on Earth was served at a place called the Coffee Connection. That was before proprietor George Howell, who fussed over his beans as if they were precious gems in a jeweler's display case, sold out to Starbucks. Frankly, I don't know how George did it. The coffee was impenetrably dark, the aroma as seductive as Sophia Loren's eyes, the taste knee-bucklingly marvelous. His shop in Harvard Square was my second office, and from there I conducted business for many years. Angels rose out of the cup, the purple clouds of dawn parted to reveal a splendid, beaming sun, and shiny brass trumpets rose to the sparkling skies and declared the commencement of the day with regal fanfare. Not the Four Seasons, not Starbucks, not even Peet's can conjure such a cup. Perhaps George Howell made a pact with the Devil; yes, the coffee was that good.

King Coffee

We are built for pleasure. Every sense we possess has the capacity to discern and appreciate it. We are meant to relish and savor the world through sight, sound, touch, smell, taste, and thought (or *insight*). Given the proper stimulus, the brain itself secretes ingenious pleasure chemicals in which our otherwise dull gray cells bathe as if in a broth of nectar. A rich cup of coffee is just such a stimulus. Coffee flings the eyes open like a window thrown up on a sunny spring day.

The reverie that a cup of hot coffee induces has captivated humanity like no other substance on Earth. For this reason, among all plants, all foods, and all drugs over time, coffee would become king. Coffee today is more widely consumed than wheat, corn, or rice and more widely traded than steel. The noble coffee bean stands at the head of the line of the psyche delicacies as the regal ruler of them all. To achieve its exalted status, coffee had to work its way into the hearts and minds of millions, insinuate itself into devious schemes, leap from country to country and continent to continent, and hold off all challengers for the caffeinated throne.

If you don't care for coffee, then by all means don't touch it. But if you do, then sip and savor without guilt or concern. For coffee is good for you, good for you, good for you, as you shall soon discover. But first, a modest account is in order of the history of mighty coffee, the noble bean, the heavenly gift that transformed the world, the strange dark brew that moves armies, drives commerce, and motivates millions every morning.

The Legend of K'hawah

Coffee is said to have been first discovered by a simple man in humble surroundings involving improbable circumstances and a group of goats. I don't know whether to believe the tale myself, but it's wonderful.

According to Middle East folklore, sometime around A.D. 850 in Abyssinia (now known as Ethiopia), a goatherd named Kaldi was tending his flock. As he was enjoying a rest in the warm sun one day, Kaldi observed his goats acting unusually lively and frolicsome. They jumped and gamboled. The goatherd was curious upon seeing this, so he paid close attention to the behavior of the frisky flock. He noticed that after eating the berries of a small tree, the goats became animated. So Kaldi ate some of the berries himself, and he felt a peculiar invigoration. He brought some of the berries back to the village where he lived, and his neighbors too enjoyed them. The people in that region made a tea-like beverage brewed from the hard green beans inside the berries. The tree was called kaffa, and the beverage made from its berries was named kaffa as well.

A couple of hundred years later, in the sparse and rugged foothills of the Yemen countryside, yet another poor goatherd tended a flock belonging to the Shehodet monastery, whose brethren worshiped Allah. The goats provided the faithful with milk, butter, meat, and leather. The goatherds of the monastery, in turn, treated the animals well, allowing them to roam and climb and frolic. By day, the goats nibbled on short grasses, sage, coltsfoot, mimosa, and caper bushes. By night, they lay down on rust-colored sands amidst dwarf acacia and slept under starry skies.

But something unknown had changed the natural habits of the flock. No longer did they calmly lie down at dusk and pass the night in peace and quiet. Instead, they scampered and bleated, leapt and ran about nervously, with no apparent need for rest. Day after day and night after night, they darted inexhaustibly to and fro. Eventually, the herdsman reported to the imam that something was not right.

The head of the monastery came to where the indefatigable goats raced and played. "What do you think is the cause of their condition?" he inquired of the goatherd. "I do not know, holy sir, but I suspect the worst—that perhaps a djinn has cast a spell upon them, and they will dance upon the Earth until they collapse and die from weariness!"

The imam had seen many things in his long years and was inclined toward practical explanations and away from supernatural causes. "This circumstance is not likely the prank of a djinn," he replied. But he was curious that the goats had barely slept in 7 days. "Tell me," the imam asked, "have these animals eaten anything out of the ordinary?" The herdsman tugged with some distress at his beard and rubbed his pate as he ruminated over the question. He did not know the answer.

The intelligent man who empties these cups of foaming coffee, he alone knows truth.

—16th-century Arabic saying

Since no solution to the vexing problem was readily forthcoming, the imam determined that they should watch the goats closely, observing everything the animals ate. "As a result of our watchfulness, the truth shall be revealed." And so, for a night and a day the imam and his assistant and the hapless goatherd paid the closest attention to the goats, where they scampered and what they ate, until the goatherd cried out in excitement, "I have found it!" In his hand he held a spray of a shrub that none of them could identify. White blossoms projected from clusters of shiny green leaves, and the plant possessed small berries with hard kernels.

The imam took the spray and turned it over and over. In all his days he had never seen such a plant. "Are you certain the goats have eaten this?" The goatherd pointed to damaged branches and places where the teeth of the animals had chewed. "There can be no doubt about it, o great sir." The head of the monastery poked at the plant, sniffed at it, and bit off a small piece of leaf, chewing it thoughtfully.

And so it was that the imam and his assistant and the goatherd collected armloads full of the newly discovered shrub, laden with its pretty flowers and strange berries. For the imam was not only learned in the teachings of the great prophet Mohammed, but he was also a man of the sciences. Back at the monastery, he would study the plant. Perhaps the same invigorating effect that overtook the goats could be felt by man.

In his chambers, the imam carefully inspected each aspect of the shrub, noting the skin of the branches, the color and shape of the leaves, the form and fragrance of its blossoms, and the peculiarness of the berries. In vessels of water he made various cold potations: one of the whole shrub, one of just the leaves, and one of just the berries, which he had crushed with a pestle. He sipped each, one at a time, and waited to notice any effect.

The imam also took the berry kernels, toasted them in a dish over a fire, and then crushed them well with a pestle. Into a small pot of boiling water he threw a generous handful of the powder. The water blackened and yielded a pleasant, nutty aroma. After consuming a cupful of the hot infusion, the imam felt strangely enlivened. Mighty Allah! he exclaimed to himself. How could a simple berry kernel be imbued with such power to stir natural vigor? The imam's mind sprang alive with exceeding wonder, as a hawk takes to flight. Ideas and thoughts arose in great profusion. The head of the monastery felt his wit quicken, as though all his senses were keener.

Indeed, never in his years had the head of the monastery come upon such a plant. So inspired was he by his discovery that the imam consulted the most learned herbalists, but none had ever heard of such a plant. Then the imam recalled something he had learned about Ethiopians who conquered Yemen centuries before. They had come from the territory of Kaffa, and among the fruits and vegetables they brought with them had been the kaffa tree.

In Damascus, Aleppo and in the residence of Cairo
It has gone round with a great Hallo!
The coffee bean, the scent of ambrosia!
Then it entered the seraglio and the air of the Bosphorus,
Seducing Doctors, Cadis and the Koran
To sects and martyrdom!—and now
It has triumphed! It supplanted
In this happy hour, in the Moslem empire,
Wine which until then was consumed!

—Belighi, Turkish poet

Now, of all the duties in a monastery, none is as wearying as the call to prayer in the dead of night. Sometimes the desperate urge to remain asleep is so overpowering that it weighs one down into a mumbling stupor. Many is the monk who has fallen down and passed out while trying to endure night prayers. Even if you can stay awake, your legs feel like wood, your arms like lead, your head stuffed with sackcloth. Anything that might improve wakefulness and ease the burden of fatigue would be a blessing.

And so, the imam had an idea. He made a strong decoction of the crushed, roasted kaffa tree berry kernels one night and, as he woke each monk for prayers, he offered a cupful of the brew: black in color, bitter in flavor, and pleasant in aroma. Each monk took the cup and drank. Instead of dragging themselves wearily out of their cells that night, the monks shed all sense of fatigue and strode to prayer awake, alert, upright, and in cheerful spirits. The monks named the drink *k'hawah*, meaning "stimulating" or "invigorating." From then on, the monks drank refreshing k'hawah together to allay fatigue.

In fact, coffee would become pervasive throughout Islam, positioned as a divine agent that not only furthered mental alertness but promoted sobriety. Islam's stance against the consumption of wine was greatly aided by the appearance of coffee. Here was a drink that worked magically upon the body and mind but in ways that furthered work and faith instead of hindering them. Coffee, the friend of the holy, would be carried like a battle flag across all of Allah's vast kingdom.

The Coffee Tree

The marvelous coffee tree makes up the genus *Coffea* in the botanical family Rubiaceae. Arabian coffee is classified as *Coffea arabica*, robusta coffee as *Coffea canephora*, and Liberian coffee as *Coffea liberica*. Varying from 6 feet to 13 feet in height, the tree is an evergreen possessed of long, slender branches covered with bright, waxy, spear-shaped leaves. It is delicate, intolerant of sudden temperature changes. Coffee flourishes at high altitudes, requires both sun and shade, needs plenty of water, must be sheltered from frost and heat exceeding 86 degrees Fahrenheit, and should be rooted in porous, well-drained soil. When all of these conditions are met, the coffee tree responds by producing a profusion of elliptic green berries that grow and ripen into bright red cherries half an inch long. The tree bears its fragrant white flowers and coffee cherries at the same time.

Inside the bright red skin of the coffee cherry is a gummy pulp that surrounds a pair of facing beans held together by a sweet parchment. These coffee cherries are picked at the peak of their redness and then processed. When only one bean is found instead of two, it is referred to as a peaberry, which some say makes a tastier coffee. Single or in pairs, coffee beans are green and waxy when pried out of their cherries. The beans are what coffee commerce is all about, because it is the bean that contains the bracing stimulant caffeine.

The simple coffee bean is a Hercules of commerce, a mighty titan that has amassed a giant workforce. It is the center of a global industry employing more than 20 million people who toil in coffee plantations, processing plants, and roasting operations.

The Three Kinds of Coffee

I remember the first time I ever stood in a coffee orchard, the first time I ever picked a ripe coffee cherry and popped it in my mouth. I was standing still amid slender trees in rural Costa Rica. Songbirds warbled and called. The sun felt warm on my neck. I had walked about a mile or so down a long, sloping mountain to a small jewel of a coffee plantation, not more than a couple of acres in all. A fastidiously neat netted shed housed the tools that kept several hundred coffee trees exquisitely well tended. I wandered through the rows. Each tree stood about 6 feet high. I picked a red coffee cherry from one of the heavy-hanging clusters and bit through the thin skin and pulp of the cherry to the two beans inside, covered with a sweet mucilage. I spat out the skin and sucked on the beans, taking in their floral sweetness. When the sweetness was gone, I spat out the beans, then plucked another, and another.

Parts of Costa Rica have the perfect conditions for growing beautiful coffee trees: year-round temperatures between 68 and 77 degrees, volcanic soil, almost daily rainfall, and an elevation of around 1,000 feet. Hundreds of coffee farms called *fincas*, many of them modest in size, produce top-quality arabica coffee beans with excellent flavor and aroma. As I stood there sampling the wares, my face broke naturally into a broad smile as I thought of the famous physician William Harvey's proclamation: "This little fruit is the source of happiness and wit!" He could have added that the coffee tree is a graceful work of nature that delights the eye as much as its fruits stimulate the body and mind.

Of the three types of coffee trees cultivated for commercial purposes, arabica is the most highly prized. According to botanical evidence, this is the variety of coffee that originated in Ethiopia and later spread throughout Islam, awakening the minds and bodies of the faithful. Arabica is the champagne of coffee. All great coffees without exception, whether from Colombia, Indonesia, Kenya, or Jamaica, are arabica beans. The beans, and the way they are roasted, convey the various flavors and aromas for which various regional coffees are known and loved. Like wine grapes, arabica beans possess the subtle flavors of the soils and environments in which they are grown, conveying rich and heavy flavors in some areas, delicate and subtle flavors in others. The arabica coffee tree requires 5 years of growth before it will produce a good yield of ripe cherries. It is less resistant to disease, especially the coffee-decimating leaf rust *Hemileia vastatrix*, than the two other commercial varieties, but if you love coffee, arabica is the only brew to consume.

Coffee, the sober drink, the mighty nourishment of the brain, which unlike other spirits heightens purity and lucidity; coffee, which clears the clouds of the imagination and their gloomy weight, which illumines the reality of things suddenly with the flash of truth.

—17th-century history book description

Like an unrefined cousin, the robusta coffee tree, which was discovered growing wild in the Belgian Congo, is less delicate than the arabica tree, producing more beans with fully double the caffeine content. Robusta beans are simply carriers for caffeine and are never noted for taste. Indeed, they taste harsh and bitter. Accordingly, they are manufactured into instant coffee and acrid canned grinds. If arabica is the champagne of coffee, then robusta is the malt liquor. A 1912 New York Coffee Exchange report described robusta as "practically worthless" due to its lousy flavor. While arabica trees are grown under specific climatic conditions, robusta trees can thrive in a wider variety of environments. The trees do well at lower elevations and are suitable for raising on hot lowland plantations subjected to temperatures that would wither arabica trees. Robusta trees produce a full crop yield in only 2 to 3 years after planting and are more resistant to disease. Despite their lack of flavor, robusta-bean coffees are very widely consumed. Highly caffeinated but flat-tasting robusta beans supply fast-food chains, diners, truck stops, doughnut shops, and supermarkets with a concentrated and fast-acting stimulant for a world on the go. Robusta coffee is a bulging biceps on the brawny musculature of the commerce of coffee, which is second only to petroleum as the most widely traded commodity in the world.

A notch below robusta on the flavor scale is liberica coffee, whose host tree is native to Liberia. Hardier and more disease resistant than arabica and robusta, liberica is the only coffee that can be grown at sea level. Yet its yields are moderate, and it is cultivated only in Liberia and parts of Malaysia, Java, and the Philippines. Liberica beans are used as filler beans in low-quality coffee blends. If arabica is the champagne and robusta the malt liquor of coffees, then liberica is the jug Tokay. Nobody chooses liberica coffee for its taste.

The Precious Beans of Kona

A warm breeze blew through open car windows as four of us cruised the Kona Coast on the western side of the big island of Hawaii. The October sun shone warmly, and the aroma of coffee roasting somewhere nearby caught my attention. "This whole area, for about 20 miles or so, is nothing but coffee," noted my friend Zachary Gibson, who rode shotgun as I drove. In the backseat, Shahannah and Zack's wife, Hanna, oohed and aahed at the sight of thousands of trees heavily laden with ripe red coffee cherries. Producing on average 10,000 pounds of ripe cherries per acre, the healthy, mature trees we saw represented a whole lot of coffee. "Look at all those," Zack called, pointing out a perfectly manicured plantation.

We had dropped onto the 20-mile-long Kona Coffee Belt at its northern end at Palani Junction and were making our way south through the heart of coffee country. Here, for more than 170 years, generations of growers have toiled to distinguish Kona as among the world's most prized coffee beans.

We admired what we could see of the 3,000 acres of coffee trees planted in the region, whose fortunes have risen and fallen like the great Pacific swells that crest and break along Hawaii's rugged coasts. In the 1950s, 6,000 acres of coffee grew on those hills, during a vigorous recovery period after a market collapse that followed an earlier coffee boom. At that time, coffee yields per acre reached an impressive 15,000 pounds. In its rising and falling, Kona's coffee fortunes were similar to those of Brazil and other coffee-producing nations. When coffee prices rise, growers plant more trees. As prices fall, trees are ripped out of the ground to reduce yields and drive up prices. In the worst cases, plantations go belly-up. Boom and bust, planting and pulling are cyclical aspects of coffee production since it became a commercial crop.

Hawaii's affair with coffee began in 1825, when the governor of Hawaii introduced coffee plants he had obtained in Rio de Janeiro. In 1828, the Reverend Samuel Ruggles, an American missionary, introduced the first coffee trees to Kona, in Naole near Kealakekua. While the first Hawaiian commercial plantings of coffee were made on the island of Kauai, coffee failed there and was replaced by sugarcane. But on the big island of Hawaii, the districts of Kona on the island's west coast and Hamakua on the east coast provided good conditions for the delicate trees. Situated between the enormous Mauna Kea volcano to the north and Mauna Loa volcano to the south, the Kona Coffee Belt lay protected from damaging winds. Additionally, Kona benefits from bright, sunny mornings and shady afternoon clouds. These atmospheric conditions, plus the volcanic soil, good elevation, and ample rainfall make Kona an ideal location for arabica-bean coffee. The multitudinous forces of nature have melded together in harmonious perfection to make for coffee an ideal home on the lush green slopes of Kona.

When world coffee prices increased in the 1890s, investors hired Chinese, Portuguese, and Japanese immigrants to work their coffee plantations in Kona. The laborers planted the trees, pruned them, picked the ripe cherries at harvest, and put their backs into creating Kona's first coffee boom. Donkeys laden with 100-pound sacks transported the ripe cherries to the coffee mills. Known as Kona Nightingales because of their loud braying, the beasts had the surefootedness and strength required to haul loads up and down Kona's steep hills.

Initially, coffee grew well in Kona, but then farmers lost crops to white scale blight. The ladybird beetle, brought from Australia in 1893, proved successful in controlling the white scale disease, and coffee plantations then thrived. While the introduction of a foreign species often results in disaster, in this case the ladybird beetle saved Kona coffee.

But by 1900, a glut of beans on the world market had led to Kona's first coffee bust. With fortunes lost, investors left the area with their pockets turned out, and Chinese and Portuguese laborers moved from the shady coffee orchards of Kona to harsh labor in the lowland cane fields. There they toiled with machetes in the broiling sun. What coffee remained in Kona was primarily cultivated by Japanese tenant farmers on small family plots. By 1910, four out of five coffee farmers in Kona were Japanese. Men, women, and their children worked side by side picking ripe cherries to deliver to either Captain Cook or American Factors, the two dominant coffee companies in that area. Coffee prices rose steadily until 1928, and the Kona farmers prospered. But the stock market crash of 1929 caused coffee prices to fall to an all-time low. Between 1930 and 1940, the number of Japanese coffee farms dropped from 1,070 to 600.

Between 1941 and 1945, the Kona coffee industry was again turned on its ear, this time by World War II, which saw many Japanese growers volunteering for military service. After the devastations and casualties of the war, however, Kona's coffee fortunes rose again with increases in world coffee prices. By 1959, 12 pulping mills operated in Kona, but then coffee prices began a giddy slide downward toward financial crisis, spelling another bust period. The Kona coffee market might have stayed down if not for the sophisticated taste of an emerging social group of gourmet coffee drinkers in the late 1970s and 1980s. The new demand for expensive, regional gourmet coffee stimulated growth and production and sent Kona coffee prices upward.

But Kona's coffee fortunes were threatened yet again, this time by an insidious force: dilution. Kona "blends" flooded the coffee market, containing as little as 10 percent real Kona coffee. Such blends, which can be found today as typically a mix of a little Kona coffee and a lot of cheap, harsh beans, diminished the fine Kona name. These coffees should rightly be labeled 90% INFERIOR BLENDS. Only a strong 100% KONA

COFFEE campaign has pulled Kona beans back up to the elevated position they so richly deserve.

There are times of great beauty on a coffee farm. When the plantation flowered in the beginning of the rains, it was a radiant sight, like a cloud of chalk, in the mist and the drizzling rain.

—Isak Dinesen, *Out of Africa*

As Zachary, Hanna, Shahannah, and I motored along, we were in search of a small plantation—and a perfect cup to boot. For this, we sought out Russell Archibald in Honaunau. We cruised up a steep drive lined on both sides by 10-foot-high coffee trees hanging heavily with green and red cherries, with some branches so laden they touched the ground. A medium-sized dog ran toward the car and barked ferociously. When we failed to respond in any way, he turned, wagged his tail, and trotted back to the house. Obviously an ambivalent watchdog, he had performed his duty and was done with the matter.

On the porch, Russell Archibald and his wife, Mickey, waved at us. He wore a bandanna, from which a braid of long gray hair ran down his back, and she sported a colorful flowy dress from another era. Their home, made of weathered wood and surrounded by a riot of flowers in bloom, conveyed a welcoming feel. They invited us in to their kitchen. There, amidst a profusion of potted plants, we sat down around a worn wooden table. "Would you folks like some coffee?" Russell inquired.

In an old grinder, Russell finely whizzed dark-roasted arabica beans from his small plantation and placed them in a cloth strainer, which he hung over a dented coffee pot. He boiled water in an old metal kettle on a gas stove and then poured it onto the coffee. Fragrant vapors steamed the air, and I leaned in to sniff. The brew was dark and strong, with a nutty cocoa aroma. Tremendous. Russell smiled warmly, and we all smiled and sat drinking lovely coffee in big cups on a warm, sunny morning on the Kona Coast.

Harvesting

Russell Archibald turned to me. "Have you ever seen coffee harvested?" I hadn't. He invited me to follow and stepped out of his kitchen and into the backyard, where he selected a woven basket from a pile of several, secured it to his waist with a belt, and headed toward coffee trees laden with red cherries. Russell explained that he grew his coffee by organic methods, without insecticides or fungicides. The trees looked healthy to me. Running his hands along the slender branches, Russell carefully plucked ripe cherries with a quick, practiced motion and laid them carefully in the basket. "This basket will hold about 20 pounds of coffee," he said. Very quickly he collected at least a pound of coffee. In the lower elevation of the 2-mile-wide Kona Coffee Belt where Russell grows his 2 acres of trees—the typical farm size in Kona—coffee cherries usually ripen and are harvested between August and February. In the cooler and wetter higher elevations of the Belt, coffee harvesting may go on all year long. A few hundred feet in elevation can make a big difference for a coffee farm.

"I used to farm vegetables," Russell commented, "but then I figured I couldn't make any money at it. I can make a little with coffee."

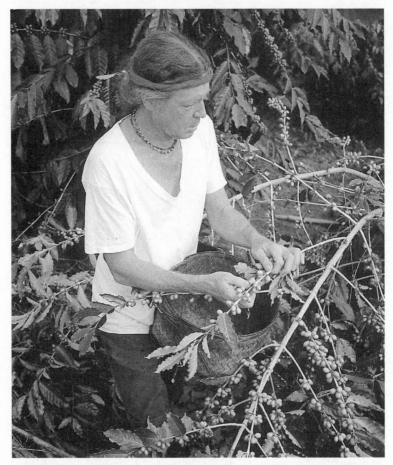

Coffee grower Russell Archibald picks precious Kona coffee beans.

Coffee is not a particularly lucrative crop even during booms, and I muse over the economics of being a grower. Approximately 6 pounds of ripe cherries result in 1 pound of green beans, which when roasted will lose 20 percent of their weight. Thus, 7.5 pounds of cherries produce 1 pound of roasted coffee. In the 2000 harvest season, growers in Kona received 75 cents per pound of cherries from processors. To gross $50,000, a Kona grower would need to harvest around 67,000 pounds of cherries.

The record harvest for an acre of Kona coffee was 19,600 pounds. But this is far from typical. According to state coffee specialists from the University of Hawaii, an average acre of mature coffee trees will yield 10,000 pounds of cherries, worth about $7,500. At those yields, a grower needs to harvest more than 13 acres of coffee to gross $100,000. That's a lot of physical labor in the heat. Plus, nobody picks that much coffee alone. An experienced picker can gather between 200 and 400 pounds of coffee cherries per day. Considering that coffee must be picked at peak ripeness and cannot be left to overripen, numerous pickers must work a farm. And the cherries do not ripen all at once. In Kona, from four to eight passes are made through a coffee plantation each harvest season. And yet hundreds of individuals like Russell Archibald, who has grown a small amount of high-quality Kona coffee for 10 years, remain devoted to the crop. Maybe a big part of that is due to the sheer beauty of the plantation—the lush green, the profusion of fragrant blossoms, the wealth of trees whose cherries yield a precious prize.

Processing

Once coffee is harvested, the grower has about 24 hours to process the cherries before they start to soften. In the first of four steps, pulping, the ripe coffee cherries are rotated in a drum and squashed. The pulp of the fruit is removed, and the coffee beans slip through grooves and are ejected out of the opposite side of the machine. The slippery coating of the coffee bean must be removed next, in a process called demucilaging. This is most often accomplished by fermenting the beans in a vat with bacteria that break down the coating until it easily dissolves in water. Then the beans are washed to remove all traces of the coating. They are now ready for drying.

Coffee beans are dried either in the sun, in mechanical rotary dryers, or on shallow drying trays that are buffeted by hot air. The beans should not be heated higher than 150 degrees Fahrenheit or they'll lose their aroma. When dried, the coffee beans still retain a parchment skin around them. In the final stage of coffee processing, the beans are milled in hulling machines. The resulting green coffee beans are ready for the process that transforms them into something holy.

Roasting

After all the work required to strip coffee beans of their many layers, you'd think they would appear special somehow. In fact, milled coffee beans offer little visual appeal. Green and waxy, they are not at all what one conjures in the mind when thinking of a steaming, fragrant cup of coffee. To become dark, aromatic, and delicious, coffee beans must be roasted. Roasting sets in motion hundreds of chemical changes inside the beans. Sugars decompose, gases are released, and a plethora of natural compounds are modified. Coffee roasting is an alchemical process by which waxy green beans are transformed into gold.

At Greenwell Farms in Kealakekua, the Greenwell family has produced high-quality Kona coffee for more than a century. Operating 40 acres of their own coffee trees and buying from hundreds of other growers in the area, Greenwell processes Kona coffee from beginning to end and sells it under its own label. Before going through their processing facilities, Shahannah, Zachary, Hanna, and I sampled several Greenwell coffees from pump thermoses. I found the peaberry and stayed with it, the perfect flavor and roast for an afternoon pick-me-up.

Emerald Freitas, whose Portuguese grandmother farmed coffee for decades in Kona, showed us around the Greenwell processing facilities. Tens of tons of coffee beans lay drying on shed roofs, and a group of men milled beans nearby. But what captured my attention most was the *fragrance* of roasting. Emerald shared some of the specifics of the delicious Greenwell roasts. "We basically have three roasts: regular, city, and dark. We roast all our beans at exactly 415 degrees. The regular roast goes for 16½ minutes, the city roast goes for 18 minutes, and the dark roast goes for 19½ minutes."

"On the nose?" I asked.

"On the nose."

Not every coffee processor is as exacting or fastidious as Greenwell, and various roasters have their preferred temperatures and times. But one thing is undeniable: The roast makes the coffee. You need great beans to yield a great coffee, but it is the roast that exalts the flavor, that produces the exotic aroma, that is tasted in the cup. Predictably, people prefer different roasts according to their taste. Some coffee drinkers like their brew on the lighter side, just as some wine drinkers prefer whites. I prefer a city roast of heavy-flavored Indonesian or African beans for a dark, ponderous cup. (And give me a rich red wine any day.)

The first coffee links me with a world I love in almost a secret way.

—Colette Modiano, *Turkish Coffee and the Fertile Crescent*

In the earlier centuries of coffee's march around the world, roasting was more often accomplished at home. In pie plates, in frying pans, or in the oven, coffee beans were heated and stirred until they evenly achieved the right color. Now, few people roast beans at home. Coffee is either roasted in giant processing facilities or in smaller, more boutique roasting operations.

So how do roasts settle out in terms of flavor?

Light roast—For delicate or mild-flavored beans, light roast is preferred by those who want coffee with a more sparing flavor.

Medium roast—The typical roast enjoyed by most American coffee drinkers results in a darker coffee with more flavor than a light roast.

Full roast—Made from a very dark bean, full roast imparts bold aroma and flavor and a very dark cup of coffee. Also called a city roast.

Very dark roast—Not a roast for a common cup, the very dark roast is reserved for espresso beans and imponderably heavy Turkish coffee, which leaves sludgy grounds at the bottom for discerning omens and signs in the thick black goo.

After the roasting comes the grading. Some Kona coffees cannot be labeled as such because they fail to conform to certain quality standards. The five grades of coffee produced in the region are Extra Fancy, Fancy, No. 1, Prime, and No. 3. These are graded according to screen size (Extra Fancy are the largest beans), cleanliness, color, moisture content, roasting quality, and flavor and aroma when brewed. No. 3 grade is inferior coffee and may not be labeled with the Kona coffee designation. Peaberries, the small, single berries that account for less than 5 percent of the total Kona coffee yield, are graded separately. Peaberries are generally more flavorful and typically command a higher price among the gourmet coffee cognoscenti.

The March to World Dominance

The history of coffee is rife with intrigue, politics, and the rise and fall of fortunes. Here are some of the highlights.

During the years between 1573 and 1578, a German physician named Leonhardt Rauwolf traveled throughout Turkey, Syria, and Persia. Along the way, he noted the natives' use of various plants and collected numerous specimens. Rauwolf wrote an account of his travels, *Reise in die Morgenlander* ("Journeys in the East"), in which he became the first Westerner to describe coffee. In the course of his explorations, Rauwolf discovered that coffee, which he found made him feel "curiously animated," was widely used throughout the region. He wrote,

> Among other things they possess a beverage which they value highly, called chaube. It is as black as ink, and very useful in various diseases, especially those of the stomach. They usually take it in the morning in public without fear of being seen. They drink it from small earthen or porcelain cups, as hot as they can bear it. They frequently lift these vessels to their lips and take small sips, and then pass them round in the order in which they are sitting. They prepare a beverage from water and a fruit which the natives call bunnu. This somewhat resembles the laurel berry in size and colour. This beverage is very much in use, and for this reason a large number of merchants may be seen in the bazaars selling the fruits or the beverage.

Rauwolf's comments on coffee stirred interest in the beverage among Europeans, who already looked to the Orient for such exotic stuffs as silks and spices. Coffee was widely consumed and traded when Rauwolf hit Asia Minor, which had a history of coffee drinking that began about 700 years prior to the good doctor's explorations. Almost certainly first consumed in Abyssinia (Ethiopia), coffee was also used in Persia in A.D. 875, according to 19th-century botanist Baron Ernst von Bibra.

From what can be pieced together concerning coffee prior to the year 1000, members of the Ethiopian Galla tribe ground up coffee beans and mixed them with animal fat. This mixture they consumed as an energy food.

Sometime around 1100, Arab traders brought coffee back to their homeland and cultivated the plant for the first time. Some historians maintain that the first coffee plantations were in Yemen, along the coast of the Red Sea. Like the Yemeni Sheikh, the Arabians found that boiling the beans was the most pleasant and palatable way to prepare coffee. This resulted in the drink they called *k'hawah*. By the late 13th century, Arabians were roasting and grinding the beans before brewing, and coffee was consumed pretty much in the form that we know today.

Coffee, you dispel the worries of the great . . . you are the drink of the friends of God . . . you are the common man's gold, and like gold, you bring to every man the feeling of luxury and nobility. You flow through the body as freely as life's blood, refreshing all that you touch.
—Sheikh Ansari Djerzeri Hanball Abd-Al-Kadir

By the time the 15th century neared its close, Moslems had introduced coffee to Persia, Egypt, Turkey, and North

Africa. Coffee became a highly prized trade item. The world's first coffee shop, Kiva Han, opened in Constantinople in 1475. At the time, it was a stunning idea. Men and women alike took to the new drink. Coffee became a regular item in the Turkish diet and a measure of marital stability: Turkish law allowed a woman to divorce her husband if he failed to provide her with her daily coffee.

Coffee faced harsh opposition in 1511, when Emir Khair Bey, the new governor of Ottoman, attempted to ban consumption of the drink. Angered that he was being lampooned by critics, the governor determined to find out about those who spoke against him. When he discovered that his detractors were all coffee drinkers, his taste for the beverage soured. He assembled a group of scholars, military leaders, and other learned men and pressed them to support his opinion against coffee. He pushed the notion that the drink was an intoxicant and as such violated the law of the Qur'an. In the end, after a great deal of wrangling, the group of scholars did declare coffee to be *mekruh*, or undesirable. But their proclamation fell far short of condemnation.

The governor was not satisfied. Stewing over the harsh jibes of his coffee-consuming critics, he ordered all coffeehouses closed, offering as his reasoning that the use of coffee led to riots. For one terrible week, coffee drinkers were abused in the most horrible ways, publicly humiliated, flogged, and driven out of town. But the Sultan of Cairo, himself an ardent coffee drinker, refused to let the order stand. He not only reversed the ban and allowed coffeehouses to reopen, but he further declared coffee to be beneficial to health and pleasing to God. This incident became pivotal in coffee's march through time and culture. News of Khair Bey's defeat spread throughout the Mohammedan world and resulted in elevated status and increased trade. Coffee had survived its first of many scrapes.

Even as coffee use boomed in the capital cities Aleppo, Damascus, and Cairo, so wine and the stores in which it was sold were driven out in the name of Mohammed. In 1554, coffeehouses opened on the Golden Horn and became known as schools of the cultured. By 1630, more than 1,000 coffeehouses operated in Cairo alone. Coffee became known as the "milk of chess-players and of thinkers." It facilitated conversation, and coffeehouses became the main places where ideas were exchanged. From the coffeepot, a great human exchange was served hot and steaming: life, religion, politics, love, art, poetry, and the sciences, virtually anything at all was fair game for hours of discussion. Coffee pried loose the conversational jaws of the east and set in motion a history-changing exchange of thought.

As long as Mocha's happy tree shall grow,
While berries crackle or while mills shall go,
While smoking streams from silver sprouts shall glide,
Or China's earth receive the sable tide,
While coffee shall to British nymphs be dear,
While fragrant streams the bended head shall cheer,
Or grateful bitters shall delight the taste,
So long her honours, name and praise shall last.
                    —Alexander Pope, English poet and satirist

From the lands of Mohammed, coffee marched mightily onward to Christendom, carried into Europe by Venetian traders. Around 1600 in Italy, Pope Clement VIII was urged by his advisers to ban coffee as an infidel threat. The pope reputedly tasted coffee to find out for himself the nature of the drink. So enamored was he of its flavor, apparently, that he chose to "baptize" coffee instead, proclaiming it to be so delicious that it would be a pity to let the infidels have exclusive use of it. Coffee, that wonder worker, had so conjured delight in the pontiff that it was assured good passage into the lives of Catholics throughout Europe. A dark and mysterious brew from the Moslem East, revered as a divine agent of sober and clear thought, soon became revered in Europe among Christians for the very same reasons. The European mind would be pried open, stimulated, and seasoned by a thousand ideological spices.

As coffee grew in popularity, intrigue surrounded its cultivation. The Arabs, protective of their precious *Coffea arabica*, refused to allow fertile seeds, coffee trees, or cuttings to legally leave their country. Transportation of the plant out of the Moslem nations was forbidden by law. But sometime around 1650, a Moslem pilgrim from India named Baba Budan snuck seven fertile coffee seeds out of Arabia. He planted his seeds in the hills in Mysore, India, where they flourished. Today, coffee trees descended from Baba Budan's smuggled beans populate the hill plantations of that region.

In 1650, a man from Lebanon named Jacobs opened the first coffeehouse in England, at Oxford. Two years later, a Greek man from Ragusa named Pascal Rosea opened the first coffeehouse in London, in Cornhill. That same year, a merchant named Edwards, who had brought coffee from the Levant (now Syria and Lebanon) and a Greek slave girl from Smyrna, opened a coffeehouse in London as well. From that point on, coffeehouses proliferated in the great city. As they spread, so did conversation and ideas. Pamphlets, leaflets, and publications of various kinds were made available in coffee-houses, and not all of them contained sentiments that were favorable to the crown. Thus, shortly before New Year's Day in 1676, England's attorney general William Jones ordered all coffeehouses closed, citing harm to His Majesty King Charles II and the realm. The resulting public outcry was so dramatic that the crown had no other option than to back down. Coffeehouses were reopened for good, and the free flow of caffeinated ideas and opinions was allowed to change the shape of England.

Coffee falls into the stomach, and there is general commotion. Ideas begin to move like the battalions of the Great Army of the Republic on the battlefield. Things remembered arrive at full gallop. . . . The light cavalry of comparisons delivers charges, the artillery of logic hurries up with trains and ammunitions, the shafts of wit start up like sharpshooters. Similes arise, the paper is covered with ink; for the struggle begins and is concluded with torrents of black water, just like a battle with powder.

—Honoré de Balzac, French novelist

Edward Lloyd's coffeehouse opened in 1688—the operation eventually became Lloyd's of London, the world's best-known insurance company. By 1700, more than 2,000 coffeehouses operated within the city. Coffeehouses were known as "penny universities," named after the charge for a typical cup of coffee. The word *tips* was coined in an English coffeehouse: A sign reading TO INSURE PROMPT SERVICE—TIPS—was placed by a cup. Those who wanted prompt service and a good seat put a coin in the cup.

The Dutch, mindful of the fact that coffee could be a lucrative crop, experimented with its cultivation using coffee plants imported from Mocca, in Yemen. In 1658, the Dutch began coffee cultivation in Ceylon (now Sri Lanka), and the Dutchman Willem van Outborn had the idea to create plantations in Java and Sumatra. The industrious Dutch also planted coffee successfully in Bali, Timor, and Celebes, establishing Indonesia as a major producer of coffee, which it remains to this day.

In Germany, coffee took off in the 1670s with the opening of the first coffeehouse in Berlin. Within 50 years, coffeehouses operated in every major German city. Coffee became tremendously popular, although some stubborn physicians claimed that the drink caused sterility. In 1732, Johann Sebastian Bach composed a humorous ode to coffee, his *Coffee Cantata*: "Ah! How sweet coffee tastes! Lovelier than a thousand kisses, sweeter far than muscatel wine! I must have my coffee. There's no way to please me except with coffee."

Coffee's arrival in Austria caused more of a stir. The Turkish army surrounded Vienna in 1683. Georg Franz Kolschitzky, a Viennese who had lived in Turkey, slipped through enemy lines to lead Polish relief forces to the city, where the Turks were defeated and fled Vienna. Among the many goods the Turks left behind were 500 sacks of "dry black fodder" that Kolschitzky recognized as coffee. He claimed the coffee as his reward for his act of bravery and opened Vienna's first coffeehouse, the Blue Bottle. In the habit of the Turks, Kolschitzky sweetened the coffee. He additionally filtered out the grounds and added milk. The resulting drink was sweet, fragrant, stimulating, and delicious. It caught on like wildfire.

Coffee inevitably spread to France, where the first coffee-house in Paris was opened in 1689 by an Italian named Francois Procope. His Café de Procope became a popular meeting place. By 1700, more than 250 coffeehouses operated in the city. French innovation changed coffee drinking forever when they made a different kind of infusion of the beverage. Up until that point, coffee was roasted, ground, and boiled. The resulting beverage was awash in grounds. By the new French infusion method, ground coffee was placed in a cloth filter over which boiling water was poured. This resulted in a cleaner, more refined, pleasant drink. The French also boiled milk and added it to coffee, making café au lait a popular breakfast beverage. Like the coffeehouses in other nations, those in France became centers for the free flow of coffee and ideas.

Coffee began its steady campaign to secure the ardent loyalty of North American colonists with the opening of the first coffeehouse in Boston in 1689. Although tea was at that time still the preferred caffeinated beverage in the new colonies, that feeling soon changed in one eruptive burst with the famous Boston Tea Party of 1773. Angry colonists, resisting a tea tax imposed by Britain's King George III, threw bales of British East India Company tea into Boston Harbor. Shunning tea became a patriotic duty. And in that shining and decisive moment in history, coffee stood proud, taken up as the national beverage in a swelling tide of patriotic fervor. Coffeehouses flourished. The coffee trade boomed. Roasting operations sprang up to meet demand. From a single Boston coffeehouse, the United States would become the greatest coffee market in the world. By the early 1940s, the coffee-powered United States imported 70 percent of the world's coffee crop.

The intrigue continued in 1714, when Louis XIV of France was made a gift of a coffee bush by the mayor of Amsterdam. The tree was lovingly cared for in the royal green-houses—and was jealously protected by its tenders. Enter Gabriel Mathieu Desclieux, a French infantry captain stationed in Martinique. Driven by a burning ambition to grow coffee on the tropical island's volcanic slopes, in 1723 Desclieux convinced the king's physician to secure for him a cutting from the precious royal coffee shrub. With his botanical treasure under glass, Desclieux boarded a ship for Martinique. Braving the attempted theft of his plant, the assault of pirates, and rough weather, the determined Frenchman brought the cutting safely to the island's lush shores.

Twenty months after stepping ashore with his prized cutting, Desclieux harvested a small crop of coffee cherries. Coffee fared well in Martinique. Fifty years later, an official survey recorded 19 million coffee trees on the island! Cultivation of the noble bean spread to Santo Domingo (now the Dominican Republic), which became for a time a major coffee-supplying nation. Mighty coffee continued to advance its standing by establishing domain in the Caribbean.

The gigantic Brazilian coffee industry also got off to an intriguing start, when in 1727 a Brazilian official named Francisco de Melo Palheta was called upon to settle a border dispute between the French and the Dutch colonies in Guiana. Not only did he accomplish the task, but he also bedded the wife of French Guiana's governor for good measure. Though the French and Dutch guarded their plantations to prevent commercial cultivation from spreading, Palheta enlisted the governor's wife's willing aid to smuggle out some coffee plants. When the good lady said good-bye to Palheta at the completion of his official mission, she presented him with a bouquet in which she hid coffee tree cuttings and fertile seeds. Palheta returned to Brazil and planted the coffee in the Para state. Once again through subterfuge, coffee had made its way to a prime growing area and taken root. Brazil would become in time the greatest coffee-producing nation in all of history.

Coffee works a miracle, sharpening the brains of the stupid. No author refreshed thereby need languish in silence. Coffee's strength and virtue double the memory. Every drop empowers us to gabble without pause, and, discarding the crutches of rhyme, to spout fable as history.

—anonymous 18th-century writer

Coffee has also contributed to the power of the military. The noble bean figured heavily in World War II, when U.S. defense workers and troops were supplied with as much coffee as they wanted. The Marines, naturally, boasted that they drank more coffee than any other branch of the service.

On the battlefront, where conditions ranged from miserable to hellish, a hot cup of coffee often provided the only warmth, comfort, and stimulation a soldier could find. Red Cross workers dispensed cups of coffee to battle-weary soldiers, and K rations included coffee as a matter of course. In fact, coffee became so associated with U.S. GIs that it became known as a "cup of Joe," referring to GI Joe, the military everyman. Patriotism, determination, superior arms, and unbending will may have won World War II, but it was coffee, black coffee, that woke soldiers up, energized them, and gave them the extra margin of strength to press on.

Today, coffee is the world's most popular beverage. Coffee beans are grown in Africa, Asia, the Caribbean, Indonesia, Oceania, and South America. The coffee-producing nations include Angola, Bolivia, Brazil, Burundi, Cameroon, Central African Republic, Colombia, Congo, Costa Rica, Ecuador, El Salvador, Ethiopia, Gabon, Ghana, Grenada, Guatemala, Haiti, Honduras, India, Indonesia, Ivory Coast, Jamaica, Kenya, Madagascar, Martinique, Mexico, Nicaragua, Nigeria, Papua New Guinea, Rwanda, Tanzania, Togo, Uganda, the United States (Hawaii), Vanuatu, Venezuela, Vietnam, and Yemen. Coffee brands such as Maxwell House and Nescafé are known around the world. And corporations like Starbucks, Dunkin Donuts, Peet's, and Seattle's Best now fight for café dominance in the United States. Coffee has spread farther and wider than any other plant, has insinuated itself into the diets and kitchens of hundreds of millions of people, and has spurred international commerce. More than 400 billion cups of coffee are consumed each year. Not bad for a bean.

Caffeine

The agent in coffee that imbues the bean with the power to march armies and mount massive commerce is caffeine, a humble alkaloid also known as 1,3,7-trimethylxanthine. In green beans, arabica coffee contains 1.1 percent caffeine by weight, liberica weighs in at a hefty 1.4 percent, and burly robusta tips the scales at 2.2 percent. Caffeine is also found in tea leaves (3.5 percent), guarana seeds (3 percent), kola nuts (1.5 percent), maté leaves (1.3 percent), and cacao beans (0.1 percent). These percentages will vary depending on varieties and growing conditions.

Whatever substance contains caffeine will be widely consumed. This is a maxim upon which you can hang your hat, assured that no philosophical or pseudoscientific wind will blow it off. Why do we consume caffeine? Because we love and crave it. And why do we love and crave caffeine? Because it makes us feel good by stimulating valuable physical and mental functions.

Brain and central nervous system (CNS)—First and foremost, caffeine stimulates the central nervous system. It enhances alertness, facilitates thought formation, and decreases mental fatigue. Simply put, it invigorates the mind.

Cardiovascular system—Caffeine stimulates the cardiovascular system and increases cardiac output.

Psyche—Caffeine inspires the weary and quickens the step of the tired.

Renal system—Caffeine is a mild diuretic.

Respiratory system—Caffeine stimulates respiration.

The caffeine contents of coffees and teas vary widely, depending on how much tea or coffee is used and the method of preparation. And caffeine consumption around the world varies too. Denmark and Sweden win top prizes for population caffeination. By contrast, consumption of caffeine in the United States is merely moderate.

As with virtually every other substance, dosage is important with caffeine. It determines whether you will have a good experience or a bad one. In this book, I am attempting to steer you toward good experiences with fundamentally safe plants, and while caffeine promotes beneficial activity in the body, too much can be a bad thing. A recent metaanalysis of caffeine studies performed at the French National Institute of Health and Medical Research concluded that at around 300 milligrams per day, caffeine improves mood, vigilance, alertness, and your overall sense of well-being. Caffeine appears to work on the dopaminergic pathway in the brain, thereby enhancing mood. For most caffeine-tolerant adults, this dosage range—two or three average-strength cups of coffee per day—produces positive effects. The caffeine content of the most popular caffeinated drinks is approximately as follows:

Brewed coffee (5 ounces): 80–175 milligrams
Percolated coffee (5 ounces): 40–170 milligrams
Cappuccino (6 ounces): 60–120 milligrams
Iced tea (12 ounces): 70 milligrams
Instant coffee (5 ounces): 45–70 milligrams
Brewed tea (7 ounces): 60 milligrams
Coca-Cola (12 ounces): 45.6 milligrams
Hot cocoa (6 ounces): 2–8 milligrams

Of course, you can consume too much caffeine. Side effects of overconsumption include nervousness, insomnia, overly rapid heartbeat, mental stress, gastric discomfort, anxiety, and tremors. The human lethal dose of caffeine is approximately 10 grams, equal to roughly 66 5-ounce cups of strong coffee. So here I must make a strong recommendation: Do not drink 66 cups of coffee. In fact, to be safe, don't even drink 50. Without question, some people do not tolerate caffeine. If you are such a type, then avoid coffee, tea, or colas. It's that simple.

Controversy surrounds the question of whether caffeine is addictive or not. In the strictest sense it may not be, but there is little doubt that caffeine users become dependent upon it for a lift. Most caffeine consumers rely on a daily dose, and many get a headache if they do not get their fix. At first blush, this may seem like proof that caffeine is addictive. But is this really that different from relying upon a certain amount of dietary fiber for proper elimination and getting constipated if you do not have it? In point of fact, we become dependent upon many things, including eating regularly, bathing, exercising, sharing the company of others, and attending religious services. One cannot reasonably make the claim that dependence alone indicates harm. It does not. I personally drink at least two large cups of coffee daily and feel pretty fantastic. Would I prefer to do without? No. Does coffee in any discernible way put me at any type of a disadvantage? No. Beware the rhetoric of dependency, for we depend on many things to make our lives comfortable.

Caution: As with all the psyche delicacies in this book, coffee is in my opinion an adults-only substance. Children's bodies are more acutely sensitive than those of adults, and coffee can exert unnecessarily aggressive effects upon their systems. As it is, children consume far too much caffeine in colas and other soft drinks. This condition can promote restlessness, nervousness, and an inability to concentrate. So, do not give coffee to your children.

Decaf: A Mistake

While some would-be coffee drinkers seek refuge in decaf, I consider this to be an unfortunate mistake. I cannot with clear conscience say anything good about decaffeinated coffee, which in my estimation is not coffee at all. Decaf does contain the same beneficial antioxidants as regular coffee, but it does not provide caffeinated coffee's splendid psyche benefits. Decaf is coffee interruptus, an aberrant human invention. It delivers a wan reminder of real coffee but without the same rich flavor and aroma and none of the satisfying stimulation. In fact, decaf drinkers actually have a higher rate of suicide than caffeinated-coffee drinkers. This is terrible, yet it does not surprise me. The denial of pleasure and stimulation can surely contribute to depression. Those who drink decaf may be more likely to take vitamins, eat cruciferous vegetables, and exercise more than regular-coffee drinkers, but such body-centered activities do not necessarily make for a healthy mind.

Still, it may interest some of you—for curiosity's sake—to learn how real coffee is ravaged into decaf. The most common method for decaffeinating coffee is direct solvent extraction. Green beans are steamed until they soften and then are flushed with the toxic solvent methylene chloride, which soaks through the beans. The solvent is extracted from the beans along with most of the caffeine. The beans are steamed again, then dried. Another method of decaffeination is the misnamed European water process, which is actually indirect solvent extraction. In this method, green beans are soaked in hot water to draw out the caffeine. This soaking also removes much of the flavor. The water and beans are separated, and methylene chloride is then added to the water to absorb the caffeine. Then the solvent is removed from the water, which still contains many of the flavor components of the coffee, and added back to the beans, returning much (but by no means all) of the flavor. The beans are then dried.

Two other methods of decaffeination that do not involve toxic chemicals are the Swiss water process and the carbon dioxide (CO_2) methods. In the Swiss process, green beans are soaked in water for several hours until 97 percent of the caffeine is removed along with most of the flavor components. The water is passed through a carbon block filter, which removes the caffeine but not the bulk of the flavor compounds. The water (and the flavor) is then added back to the beans, and the beans are dried. In the CO_2 method, green coffee beans are moistened with water and put into a vessel that is then filled with pressurized carbon dioxide, which draws out the caffeine from the beans. In a separate vessel, the caffeine precipitates from the CO_2, which is then cycled back into coffee. When the beans are rendered 99.9 percent caffeine-free, the CO_2 circulation is stopped and the coffee is dried to about the original moisture content. Finally, mercifully, the poor beans are ready for roasting.

The "New" Coffee

You stroll into any one of the cafés that are popping up like weeds through sidewalk cracks, look at the mini menus posted overhead or chalked in longhand on blackboards, and say to yourself, What the heck is a machiatto? Why do these people say "venti" instead of "big"? Gone, it seems, are the days when you could simply order a cup of regular coffee.

Like it or not, trendy café culture is here to stay. Luckily, most of these places happen to serve some pretty good coffee. So, if you are going to survive in the new world order without being marked as a rube, you need to know the lingua café. Sit up straight and pay attention; here is a brief primer to the first wave of designer coffees.

Espresso. Finely ground dark roasted coffee is infused with pressurized steam, resulting in a 1½-ounce serving of concentrated, intense flavor. This is not your Big Gulp cup; it is a shot. A **doppio** is a double.

Cappuccino. Espresso topped with foamed milk. Comes in a bigger cup than an espresso but contains the same diminutive serving of coffee. You can get a double, but only if you ask politely.

Latte. Got milk? Here we have a shot of espresso mixed with a big load of steamed milk and topped with a layer of milk foam. Call it a Way Milky.

Espresso machiatto. A shot of espresso with a fine layer of milk foam on top. Truly effete, and too little of anything for my taste.

Caffe Americano. Espresso with milk added to the dilution of regular coffee. Why not have a nice cup of good drip grind instead? Mysterious.

Café Cubano (Miami customers). A shot or two of espresso, with enough sugar to melt your teeth on the spot. Very strong, very sweet.

Cup of coffee. Hard to find. Confuses the help when you ask for it. Instead, try "Cuppa caffea" or "Venti doppio caffea," and you might actually get what you're after. Or, be bold and make up your own café lingo. They do.

Just Plain Good for You

As we have seen, not all people throughout history have reveled in coffee's popularity or believed in its beneficial effects. As is true for any popular celebrity, coffee has had its share of detractors. Ever since Khair Bey's short-lived ban on coffee in 1511, the beverage has been criticized by some as injurious to health.

A purportedly authoritative paper presented to faculty physicians at the University of Marseilles in 1679 declared that burned particles in coffee "sweep along all the lymph . . . and drain the kidneys." Furthermore, the paper claimed, "The ash contained in coffee induces such persistent wakefulness that the nerve fluid dries up; when it cannot be replaced, general prostration, paralysis, and impotence ensue." In 1715 France, coffee was "proven" to shorten life. Later, the beverage was said by physicians to cause inflammation of the liver and spleen.

The father of homeopathic medicine, German physician Samuel Hahnemann, fretted in 1803 that coffee produced "a wakefulness wrested from nature." He believed that by dispelling morning sluggishness and grogginess quickly, coffee produced an "artificial sprightliness" that was somehow disadvantageous to the human organism. A century later, American cereal manufacturer C. W. Post concurred. The flamboyant Post called coffee a "drug drink" and tried to scare people off it. In 1910, print ads for his bland-tasting grain beverage Postum warned that "coffee wrecks some persons." Since that time, various health food gurus including Paul Bragg, Gaylord Hauser, Bernard Jensen, and Paavo Airola have eschewed coffee, describing it variously as unhealthful, toxic, poisonous to the system, and so on. To this day, health articles and books rage against this beverage, and fanatic food faddists recommend alternative concoctions made of roasted barley and chicory as a way to kick a coffee "addiction."

So it comes as no surprise that people often express guilt over consuming coffee. Maybe you yourself have fallen victim to this miserable form of oppression. It is time now to fight back with dignity and honor. Let us with sober minds consider the unexpurgated, scientifically scrutinized, true lowdown on coffee, without vagary, mumbo jumbo, fanaticism, knee-jerk reactionary hysteria, deception, or pseudoscience.

First of all, let's wrestle to the ground the oft-repeated historical claim that coffee promotes sterility, impotence, loss of libido, or some other manner of erotic withering. For example, an account of travels in Persia by Adam Olearius in 1635 describes the effect of coffee as "to sterilize nature and extinguish carnal desires." About 40 years later, unhappy that their husbands spent more time in the coffeehouses than at home, a group of women railed against coffee in London. A poster printed in the city stated the following:

> The Women's Petition Against Coffee Representing to publick consideration the grand inconveniences accruing to their SEX from the excessive use of that drying, enfeebling LIQUOR. Presented to the Right Honorable the Keepers of the Liberty of VENUS.

In truth, coffee does not cool ardor, lower one's staff, defuse seed, or dry the body's viscid, lusty juices. Sure, if you down a gallon of potent coffee all at once, you may be too jittery to engage in lovemaking, but technically coffee does not harm your libido or sexual function. To the contrary, a well-timed cup of coffee can banish the fatigue of a wearying day and perk you up for amorous activity.

Within the previously stated dosage range of 300 milligrams of caffeine per day (typically two or three cups), coffee improves the negative moods that sometimes fog the mind upon rising. Coffee, as the most flavorful and potent caffeine-bearing beverage of all, increases general happiness and feelings of pleasure and promotes an upbeat, positive sense of self and an overall feeling of well-being. This is why people love coffee so. Baron Ernst von Bibra referred to coffee as a "pleasure drug." He hit the nail right on the head. Simple, cheap, easy to prepare, readily available, and fast acting, coffee simply makes you feel good.

Coffee even appears to reduce the risk of Parkinson's disease. Coffee drinkers have between three and six times lower risk of developing Parkinson's as compared with non–coffee drinkers. The reduction in risk generally improves as consumption increases.

O Coffee! You, friend of Allah, dispeller of sorrow! You provide health, wisdom, and truth, and you resemble gold because wherever you are obtainable the best of men will be found!
—Sheikh Ansari Djerzeri Hanball Abd-Al-Kadir

Research into the natural chemical properties of coffee shows that the daily brew is a potent protective potion. Over the past decade or so, the scientific literature has been flooded with significant studies showing that certain substances in foods called polyphenols promote antioxidant activity. To put it simply, antioxidants inhibit the rusting of cells in the body. Just as metals rust due to exposure to oxygen, so too cells in the body become damaged by exposure to certain reactive oxygen species. Oxidative damage is associated with diabetes, arthritis, cancer, degenerative brain disorders, and numerous aspects of aging and degeneration. Antioxidants found in foods—such as beta-carotene, selenium, and vitamins C and E, among others—help prevent this cellular damage, thereby reducing the risk of some diseases and extending cell life.

Coffee is, in fact, a polyphenol elixir and is especially high in one group of antioxidants called flavonoids. These compounds exhibit protective power against cardiovascular disease by reducing the oxidation of LDL cholesterol, the so-called bad cholesterol. By inhibiting oxidation of LDL cholesterol, coffee helps to protect against atherosclerosis, heart attack, and stroke.

Nevertheless, some concern has been voiced about coffee and its effects upon heart health. Here again, the news from the scientific and medical sector is good. Large-population studies suggest that coffee does no harm to the heart and does not increase the risk of any cardiovascular disease when consumed in moderation. This is even true among individuals who consume six or more cups daily. But I do not recommend that high intake, due to the nervousness that may ensue.

When properly prepared, coffee does not raise serum cholesterol. Coffee made by the drip method or by percolation has little or no effect on serum cholesterol levels. Boiled and unfiltered coffee, however, has been shown to increase cholesterol levels among coffee-drinking individuals in the Netherlands. Your best bet for the heart-healthiest cup is filtered coffee. Nor does coffee elevate blood pressure in regular coffee drinkers. Major epidemiological studies show no correlation between coffee consumption and hypertension.

The same is true for cardiac arrhythmia. While excessive coffee intake may set the heart fluttering, moderate coffee consumption does not cause irregular or rapid heartbeat.

On the other hand, the effects of coffee on the digestive system are relatively well known. Coffee stimulates gastric secretion, and for this reason a cup after lunch or dinner may help digest the meal. The morning cup of coffee not only awakens the body and mind but stimulates bowel activity as well. A strong cup increases peristalsis, the wavelike motion of the intestines that stimulates intestinal elimination. Many people rely on this action. While coffee shouldn't substitute for a healthy amount of fiber in your diet, its contribution to proper intestinal elimination is something to consider.

Coffee not only works as a laxative, it also plays a role in preventing some serious digestive disorders. Drinking two or three cups of coffee a day can reduce your risk of developing gallstones by as much as 40 percent. Coffee consumption also shows a strong protective effect against cirrhosis of the liver. Daily intake of three or four cups of coffee can reduce the risk of cirrhosis by as much as 80 percent. It can also help ease asthma and can even aid in weight loss.

If you worry that drinking coffee is going to cause some form of cancer down the line, you can relax. Again, the reported news is good news. Several major studies have failed to show any link between coffee consumption and prostate, breast, pancreatic, or bladder cancers. Nor has any link been firmly established between coffee consumption and fibrocystic breast disease. Simply put, coffee consumption is not known to increase the risk of any type of cancer. In fact, coffee exhibits a protective effect against colon and rectal cancers, reducing the risk by as much as 24 percent.

What about your bones? It is true that caffeine has a negative effect on calcium absorption. One study has found that women who consume more than 817 milligrams of caffeine per day—more than six cups of medium-strength coffee—are at three times greater risk of suffering hip fractures than women who consume no caffeine. But other studies show that moderate consumption of coffee is not associated with bone loss, increased risk of osteoporosis, or higher rates of bone fractures. The message of the studies seems clear: With moderate consumption, coffee has no negative effect upon bone health.

Women have long felt concern over their consumption of coffee and its effects on fertility, pregnancy, and a possible increased risk of miscarriage or birth defects. So far, studies do not show any link between coffee and decreased or delayed fertility. There is no evidence of increased risk of miscarriage as a result of moderate coffee consumption, nor any known association with either delayed fetal growth or increased rates of birth defects. In other words, a woman can enjoy a moderate amount of coffee daily and still become pregnant and give birth to a healthy baby.

Even athletes, who traditionally eschew coffee, may think again. A few studies have shown that caffeine actually enhances the body's ability to burn body fat. A cup of coffee before working out can do you good by enhancing both performance and endurance.

In the end, coffee's most profound effects are exerted upon the brain and mind, for coffee is the great, bold awakener. As a caffeinated beverage, coffee supercharges the brain, facilitating cognitive function overall. It stimulates the flow of blood, increases secretion of the important feel-good neurotransmitter serotonin, and otherwise invigorates the mind. It enhances alertness and motivation, facilitates thought-formation and concentration, and decreases mental fatigue. Coffee rouses the mental faculties as surely as streaming sunshine and melodious birdsong awaken the sleeping.

The Search for the Perfect Cup

If you wish to experience what I truly believe to be the perfect cup of coffee, you must travel to Caracas, Venezuela. There, in the Altamira section of that bustling equatorial city, French-Canadian Jean Paul Coupal runs Arabica Café and Café Coupa. To say that Coupal is a fanatic doesn't begin to describe the level of vigor he brings to coffee. Jean Paul Coupal combines unbridled fanaticism with a quick and brilliant mind, an apparently insatiable appetite for knowledge, a willingness to go to extremes, an obsessive sense of absolute perfection, and an infectiously delightful manner of speech and behavior, all fused together in his passion for coffee. It takes but 1 brief hour in his all-consuming company to recognize that Jean Paul Coupal is the Leonardo da Vinci of coffee.

"I have figured that there are a minimum of 120 steps from the plantation to the final roast in which coffee quality can be maintained or degraded," Coupal explained, the fever of his coffee-zealous aura heating the side of me near him. "I've also figured how to control every single one of them. It's an extraordinary task, but it's the only way to guarantee absolutely perfect coffee, from cultivation to roasting and preparation." But I was only partly listening. Most of me was otherwise engaged in the soaring, divine experience of enjoying a cup of his espresso. A layer of foamy *crema* in my cup—the result of perfect steaming—looked like milk. But in fact it was all coffee, the sign of an exquisite cup, one whose bitterness is muted and delightful, a cup whose flavors and aromas dance all over the tongue and ping against the olfactory bulb, a swooning cup, the Mozart of cups, a cup that can pick you up and dance you down the street and into the hills. I told myself that I must pay attention because the master was speaking.

I often marvel at the intricacies of other people's life paths. When Jean Paul Coupal first drank Venezuelan coffee, it so impressed him that he set out to discover the various *fincas* in that country. The only way he could manage the task was to travel to Europe and chase down the former buyers of coffee from Venezuela's Blohm & Abbott, who had once exported coffee to Europe. Going through old files from coffee purchasers, Coupal found bills of lading that identified the Venezuelan growers who used to supply Blohm & Abbott. Coupal established contact with those growers—who were still in business—and his heroic march toward coffee perfection began.

"Thanks to government intervention in the coffee industry, Venezuelan coffee quality has plummeted over the last 30 years," Coupal explained. "The government has pushed a low-grade robusta/arabica blend that's very high-yield. And this has degraded Venezuelan coffee. It's such a shame, because Venezuela is home to some extraordinary bourbon criollo single varieties of coffee. These are the only coffees I'll use. I'll put these coffees up against beans from anywhere."

Coupal's Arabica Café has been open since 1991, a shrine to the highest coffee art. Inside, a gleaming Probat roaster dominates a quarter of the floor space. Near the front window, a UNIC espresso machine sits like a buddha in a stupa. "This machine is the Rolls-Royce of coffeemakers," Coupal told me. "It's made in Nice, France, by a bunch of Italians, and nobody makes a machine that even comes close. It's the only machine I would use here." Described by France's national newspaper *Libération* as "the man who wants to be coffee king of Venezuela," Coupal has established Arabica Café as a bastion of coffee excellence and the front line against coffee mediocrity. Antique Yemeni brass coffeepots line shelves.

Coffee-themed artwork from around the world adorns the walls. Turkish-made glass apothecary jars with brass tops display single estate and single variety coffees.

"Coffee is like wine," Coupal said. "You have a cabernet grape grown in a certain valley and made into wine by a certain winery, and it has particular characteristics. The same is true with coffee. Beans from one plantation will differ from beans from another. If you control all the quality steps and roast each bean to best bring out its own unique flavors and aromas, you get exquisite coffee." I could not argue any of it. Lifting the brass tops of one jar after another, I hovered above each, taking in the aromas of coffees from fincas named La Estancia, La Hacienda, and La Orchieda.

A cup of coffee is a miracle. A miracle like a musical harmony, a wonderfully compounded assemblage of relationships.
—H. E. Jacob, *Coffee: The Epic of a Commodity*

Jean Paul Coupal has started a modest but potent coffee revolution in Venezuela. Beginning with only 2 *fincas*, he now obtains coffee from 18. The coffee cognoscenti flock from literally all over the world to Arabica Café to marvel at this mecca and to drink this perfect coffee. Coupal has been written up in dozens of magazine articles. People send him their credit card numbers, ask him to ship them coffee, and never ask the price. The list of celebrity chefs, gourmands, food writers, entertainers, and government officials who make the pilgrimage to Arabica Café would comprise an impressive volume of *Who's Who*.

Coupal's successful roasting business, Café Coupa, serves offices, hotels, and restaurants. His volume of production is significant enough that it has revived both traditional basket weaving on coffee plantations and a sisal-bag factory. In the case of baskets, Coupal insists that all coffee picked for his enterprise must be put into woven, natural fiber baskets instead of plastic pails. This edict has given new life to a dying art and now provides a livelihood for numerous women artisans. In the case of the sisal bags, Coupal was unwilling to use the normal woven bags whose fibers are impregnated with petroleum oils. Rather, he restarted Sisal Tex in Barquisimeto, Venezuela, which lubricates its fibers only with vegetable oils. "You have to control everything," Coupal declared. "It all makes a difference."

Sitting in front of Arabica Café on a warm, moderately humid equatorial morning, I sipped a tall café negro with perfect crema. Puffy white clouds chugged across a blue sky. A slight breeze stirred the leaves of nearby trees. A pair of vultures, as elegant as any birds in the air, rode a thermal over a high building without flapping a wing, and disappeared. I sipped slowly, letting the cup linger at my lips, allowing the aroma to waft upward into my nose. The exquisite grace of the moment overtook me, suffused as I was with reverie.

Chocolate
Food of the Gods

Two weeks before Christmas, La Praline Chocolatier was packed with eager customers. They pressed closely toward shiny display cases, eyes glassy with desire, biting their lips for self-control. Men jingled change in their pockets and tapped their shoes on the marble floor. Women pulled absently at their hair and worried the straps of their handbags. The atmosphere was urgent with yearning and anticipation, prickly with ardor for chocolate. My friend Craig Weatherby and I took in the marvelous scene in the company of K. C. Miller, export manager for Chocolates El Rey, manufacturer of arguably the finest chocolate in the world. "You have to meet Ludo," K.C. had told us beforehand. "He uses only El Rey chocolate, and his shop is the best I've ever seen."

Indeed, it was like a trip to Oz. Situated in the Altamira district of Caracas, Venezuela, not very far from the Arabica Café, La Praline Chocolatier is a monument to the high art of chocolate, proof that mortal humans can, by the labors of their own hands, ascend to divine heights with materials from the Earth. Glistening glass cases held fantastic displays of mouthwatering bonbons of every size and description. Plates were piled high with cups, squares, truffles, pralines, bark, stars, hearts, trees, angels, clogs (yes, the shoes), and houses made of dark chocolate or milk chocolate, many filled with nuts, creams, nougats, and mousses. A chocolate lover could go mad here. If there is a chocolate shop in Heaven, it is modeled after La Praline.

In the center of the room, behind the case, a slender, handsome man wearing glasses and a welcoming smile stood in a chocolate-stained white apron. Around him, a dozen women fussed over holiday boxes for customers. Ludo Gillis, master chocolatier, wore the smile of a happy man who has attained consummate mastery over his craft. He alertly surveyed the crowd of eager customers as individuals took their turns at the counter, selecting a dozen of this, and six of that, and well, why don't I just take a few of those over there, as long as I'm here. He smiled warmly as the patrons received their chocolates and held the boxes close, hugging the fruits of his labors like babies.

The walls of La Praline display cacao art, photographs of chocolate making, and shelves of artifacts and memorabilia such as old chocolate tins and cocoa cups. On the floor against one wall sat an old stone chocolate mill with heavy granite rollers, used to grind cacao beans into a fine paste. Brilliant recessed pinpoint halogen lights glistened like stars from the ceiling. The mood was festive—extraordinary. Bustling around the register and from one part of the shop to another, Ludo's wife, Lisette, briskly took care of business. She and Ludo both looked remarkably happy. "Pretty amazing, huh?" K.C. asked. Craig and I both admitted that we had never seen a place like it. What a spectacle. The air was suffused with complex chocolate smells, a troupe of chocolate ballet dancers performing *The Nutcracker* on my olfactory organ.

"My God," Craig let out, surveying the delights in the cases. "This is unbelievable."

Ludo spotted K.C. and walked over to greet his old friend. We made introductions all around, and Craig and I complimented Ludo on the extraordinary display. Ludo, we discovered, was a man who spoke sparingly and let his chocolates do all the bragging. He ducked away for a moment and returned with a small silver tray of oblong truffles in the shape of cacao pods, covered with a thick dusting of cocoa powder. Ludo gestured with his chin for us to try them. I selected one and bit through a thick, crunchy, semisweet dark chocolate shell into a smooth, creamy dark chocolate mousse. Tears welled in the corners of my eyes, and I looked up at Ludo, who acknowledged with a warm smile. "Good, eh?" He raised an eyebrow. Good? No. *Colossal, triumphant, majestic, lofty, inspired, sacred, fiendish, ravishing, captivating.* I swooned. My knees went weak. It was, quite simply, the very best piece of chocolate I have ever put in my mouth, and I shall never forget it.

We talked chocolate, and Ludo took us on a tour of the inner sanctum, the large kitchen where he and his wizardly staff of chocolatiers turn out the finest bonbons on earth. Pots of chocolate sat warming on stoves. Trays of cocoa powder were spread out on large tables. Bonbons of all sizes and shapes lay in various stages of assembly around the kitchen. K.C. told us that government ministers and visiting dignitaries make a point of stopping in at La Praline anytime they can. "They might miss an appointment, but they will never miss a trip to this shop."

We watched a young man and woman carefully roll small logs of soft, warm, dark chocolate in cocoa powder. That necessitated trying them, and they were marvelous beyond description. Holding up a hand, Ludo pinched the tips of his fingers together to describe something essential. "We really do try to make the very best chocolates here. This way, we are satisfied with our work, and our customers are happy."

Near the end of our visit, after we had joined the crowd and purchased our own boxes of world-class bonbons, Ludo offered another small silver tray, this one with coffee-filled dark chocolate squares. "Try one of these." Craig, K.C., and

I selected one each and bit in. Simultaneously, we burst out laughing, overtaken by sheer, unrestrained pleasure.

Melts in Your Mind, Not in Your Hand

Mysterious and exotic gift from the ancient Maya, chocolate promotes a luxurious, content mood and inspires a serene sense of sumptuous delight. Its rich flavor, silky feel in the mouth, and earthy aroma have captured the palates and imaginations of people for more than 3,000 years. Throughout history, lovers have turned to chocolate as an aphrodisiac. The Aztec emperor Montezuma reportedly downed a large goblet of chocolate drink before retiring to his harem. In the same way, the legendary Italian seducer Giovanni Giacomo Casanova reputedly consumed chocolate before bedding his lovers, a sport he engaged in with tremendous vigor and frequency, if historical accounts are even half accurate. Scientific discoveries regarding chocolate's love-enhancing components only further bolster the amorous reputation of this blissful food of the gods.

A growing body of formal research has revealed to some modest extent how and why chocolate promotes such pleasure. Chocolate is a Trojan horse, carrying into the body many hundreds of natural compounds, some ordinary and some exotic, which work busily to modify mood in subtle yet undeniable ways. One of the many compounds in chocolate is phenethylamine, or PEA. This chemical, which occurs in small quantities in chocolate, stimulates the nervous system and triggers the release of pleasurable opiumlike compounds known as endorphins. It also augments the activity of dopamine, a neurochemical directly associated with sexual arousal and pleasure. Phenethylamine floods the brain during orgasm, and more generally when we are in love, triggering that giddy, restless feeling. This fact adds a rather remarkable dimension to the appreciation of chocolate and may account for why it is so highly prized. For while there are a great many agents in nature that boost libido and enhance sexual function, chocolate alone actually promotes the brain chemistry of being in love. For this reason, chocolate is the gift of lovers.

Chocolate further boosts your sense of well-being by increasing levels of the feel-good brain chemical serotonin, which, when secreted in the right amounts, can also prevent depression and enable a good night's sleep. Thus, chocolate provides a highly desirable mood boost to women during PMS and menstruation, when serotonin levels are often down due to the neurochemical changes that occur as a result of normal hormonal fluctuations. In fact, women are consistently more sensitive to chocolate than men, and they typically experience stronger chocolate cravings. (The antidepressant drug Prozac also boosts brain levels of serotonin, but Prozac is notorious for deadening libido; better to get your mood lift from love-promoting chocolate!)

I think that you could call chocolate a soft drug. It definitely has an effect on your brain chemistry, on your physiology. I think that a lot of chocolate consumption is based on an individual's need to self-medicate. They feel a need to have a certain amount of chemicals in their brain soup, in their cranium, and chocolate does that.

—Timothy Moley, chocolatier

Another constituent of chocolate that alters mental state in pleasurable ways is anandamide, whose name derives from the Sanskrit word *ananda*, which means bliss. Anandamide is a cannabinoid, a member of the same psychoactive family of substances found in cannabis. Anandamide binds to the same receptor sites in the brain as THC, the active mind-altering molecule in cannabis. And its effect? Anandamide produces a global feeling of euphoria. This compound may account for why some people become euphoric or blissed-out when they eat chocolate. The brain is a deep and mysterious organ whose dark folds and gray crenellations are barely understood. But tickle the right neurons, and all heaven breaks loose.

Some scientists question whether there are sufficient quantities of either PEA or anandamide in chocolate to produce euphoria in humans. Of course they question—that's their job. But there are plenty of true believers. Why would chocolate develop a long-standing reputation for enhancing mood if it had no effect? Body chemistry appears to be key to how individuals react to chocolate, as is the case with almost everything. Chocolate may have little impact on some people even while it makes others swoon. So-called chocoholics may experience overwhelmingly powerful cravings and also a commensurate radical mood shift when they eat some. My mother is a case in point. Leave her in a room with a Whitman's Sampler and she'll polish off the whole box—and it stones her like a big joint of Acapulco Gold. To many, chocolate is an agent of fine and lovely reverie, a gift that allows us to reflect on our highest selves.

Cacao and the Creation

It is not easy being the Creator. There is a huge amount of work to do and no reliable help. If you want to get anything useful done, you have to do it yourself, and sometimes the work must be done over and over until you get it right. Thus, it was no easy matter when Heart of Sky, as the Maya call their Creator, decided to make human beings. Some say this occurred overnight, but don't you believe it. A piece of work as magnificent as a human being takes time and energy to create.

According to the Popol Vuh, the Mayan book of creation, Heart of Sky determined that he wanted to make a being that would worship him through speech and thought. At that time there was only the sky, and the sky couldn't praise his glory and greatness. He figured that the being should stand on solid ground. So he spoke the word "Earth," and the Earth formed. Encouraged by his success, Heart of Sky said, "Mountains," and great mountains arose. He said, "Trees," and vast forests sprang up. Indeed, his work was moving along at quite a fast pace. Then Heart of Sky imagined the various creatures of the forest and the sea, and quite quickly, the entire world was teeming with birds and fish and deer and jaguars and snakes and insects and all manner of living things swimming, crawling, slithering, walking, and flying. He felt pretty good about himself, and who could blame him?

Heart of Sky was on a roll, so he commanded the various creatures to praise him. But they only squawked, hooted, chirped, growled, barked, and made other noises. This was not the kind of glad, glorious, and intelligent praise the creator had in mind. So Heart of Sky fashioned a being out of mud, with arms and legs and a head. But the creature crumbled and fell apart. Not only did the creature not praise him, the creature didn't even hold together.

So Heart of Sky got the idea to fashion a being out of wood. "This will hold together," he said to no one in particular in a loud, godly voice. The being held together all right, but it was as dumb as a stump. Heart of Sky then tried fashioning a being out of stone. Another mistake. It, too, stayed together but did not utter even a faint murmur of praise.

So, contrary to some reports, it took a whole heck of a lot longer than a day or a week to make humans.

Finally, at one point, Heart of Sky had a brilliant idea, the kind of breakthrough idea that only a truly creative Creator can conceive. For his next attempt he selected an inspired mix of raw materials from nature: water and earth and wood and maize and cacao and numerous fruits, large and small. This time, glory be on high, it worked. Not only did the creature stay together, but it grew and thrived. And best of all, when Heart of Sky commanded the creature to praise him, it did.

So it came to pass that cacao was one of the essential materials used by the god of all Mayan gods to create human beings. And as is only right for a plant of such importance to our very being, cacao has been held in the utmost esteem from that day onward.

Cacao the Plant

Southwest of Caracas, K.C., Craig, and I motored along in tropical heat through the lush green Venezuelan countryside, past Caucagua and Panaquire to El Clavo, a picturesque rural town. There along the lazy, muddy Rio Chico, we pulled up to La Concepción plantation. Even though Africa is the world's largest producer of cacao, the fruit from whose seeds chocolate is made—Africa's gigantic 1-million-ton annual harvest dwarfs Venezuela's 14,000 tons—this South American country's cacao remains unsurpassed for quality. Craig and I were eager to see the 98-year-old plantation, home of Carenero Superior, a special hybrid of cacao.

At the gate of La Concepción we were greeted by the manager, Arsenio, who runs the plantation for owner Silvino

Reyes. We set off by foot toward what seemed like endless acres of glistening green cacao trees. "We have 176,000 cacao trees here," Arsenio explained, waving his machete in a semi-circle as we maneuvered our way along a muddy track made gooey by drenching rains the night before. "Most are Ca-renero Superior, but we also have some young Porcelano trees, and even a few Wasaré, the mother cacao." K.C. ex-plained that the strains of cacao cultivated at La Concepción produced extraordinarily flavorful and aromatic chocolate—the only kind he'll export for Chocolates El Rey.

The rainforest tree from which chocolate originates is *Theobroma cacao*, which owes its name to the 18th-century Swedish botanist Carolus Linnaeus. The Latin binomial means "food of the gods," as apt a moniker as could possibly be as-signed. There is dispute among experts regarding the origin of the cacao plant. Some say it comes from the Orinoco Valley of Venezuela, some say the Brazilian Amazon, and some con-tend that it is native to Central America. The various experts base their claims on historic use of cacao throughout time.

But new genetic testing may settle the argument. Ac-cording to El Rey owner Jorge Redmond, DNA sampling shows that the original cocoa beans—to be clear, the *cacao* tree produces seeds that are known as *cocoa* beans—migrated to Mexico from Venezuela's Maracaibo basin. Redmond holds that the *criollo* type beans were carried by Indians from the Maracaibo region. At a later point in time, Spanish priests os-tensibly brought that bean back to the northeastern coast of Venezuela to plant on plantations. In Venezuela, the Spanish found that they were having problems with plagues, bugs, and blights. Consulting with cacao experts at that time, the Spanish decided to hybridize the aroma and flavor of the criollo type of cacao with the productivity and resistance of *forastero*, another variety. This resulted in the *carenero* variety of cacao, probably in the early 1700s. This robust bean possessed wonderful flavor and aroma, which became characteristic of Venezuela's highly regarded chocolate.

The intriguing DNA findings and the historic account espoused by Redmond must wend their way through the botanical community before they are universally accepted. If and when that happens, then Venezuela will be identified as the spot where the food of the gods first sprang forth in nature.

While *Theobroma cacao* may grow appreciably taller in the wild, the cultivated tree ranges between 12 and 27 feet in height. The cinnamon brown trunk usually does not exceed 6 feet in length. The branches of the cacao tree are covered with shiny, dark green leaves about 10 inches long and 3 inches wide. Though the tree bears fruit and flowers year-round, usually there are two harvest seasons for gathering the fruit. The actual months of harvest will vary somewhat depending upon the location of the plantation.

Cacao trees bear clusters of pale, button-sized, five-petaled, faintly scented flowers growing off the trunk and

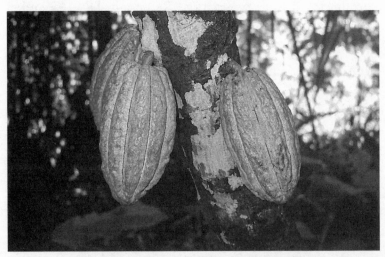

Cacao fruits ripen on a Venezuelan plantation.

bigger branches. The large, distinctive fruit pods of the tree jut out directly from the trunk and the lower branches. Young fruit pods tend to be greenish in color, but as they mature over the course of 5 or 6 months, they become elliptical in shape and bright red or yellow. The fruit pods average about 9 inches in length and typically contain between 30 and 40 almond-sized seeds (what we know as cocoa beans) nestled in a pale white flesh. It is these seeds that are made into the heavenly food loved around the world.

Cacao trees are adaptable to a wide range of moisture conditions. They can grow from tropical (very wet) to subtropical (drier) zones, but they do require fairly consistent temperature for healthy growth, with a recommended mean of 79 degrees Fahrenheit. Cacao tolerates wind and thrives best in high humidity and rainfall and deep, well-drained soil. On plantations, cacao trees can be spaced as closely as 8 feet apart. The tree is tolerant of shade and does not mind company, so cacao is often intercropped with banana, rubber, coconut, or oil palms.

Though cacao originated from either South or Central America, the tree is now cultivated in virtually every tropical area in the world. Cacao is grown commercially throughout Central and South America, the Caribbean, Africa, Indonesia, Malaysia, and the Pacific islands. This widespread distribution is testimony to the popularity of the tree and the blissful fruit from which chocolate is made.

Cacao Varieties

The three varieties of *Theobroma cacao* are criollo, forastero, and *trinitario*. Some botanists believe that at one point in time, wild cacao was distributed from Mesoamerica to the Amazon basin, and that disease eventually wiped out populations of cacao between the two areas. This, they say, resulted in two distinct varieties, criollo and forastero. The Mesoamerican criollo bears longer, pointed pods with deep ridges and white seeds. The South American forastero variety bears a rounder, more melonlike pod with purplish seeds.

The criollo variety of cacao produces a bean with more sophisticated flavor. Its downside is that the plant itself is delicate and sensitive to variations in climate and atmosphere. By contrast, the less flavorful forastero variety is more prolific and thrives in more variable conditions. Inevitably, the two were cross-pollinated, resulting in the hardy and flavorful trinitario variety. Numerous strains of each variety have been bred and refined, and certain plantations have trees whose fruits bear more flavorful cocoa beans than others.

Harvest Time

Jesús Alliendres is manager of Agropecuaria San José, an outfit that buys and sells cacao in the area outside of Carupano, Venezuela. He, Craig, and I sped along rutty roads in a Chevy pickup truck, blowing a thick, cloudy stream of road dust as we passed through sleepy Rincon. Our destination was a plantation in rural El Pilar in Sucré state. There on the edge of a vast, swampy delta, the harvest was on amidst the plantation's 275,000 cacao trees. "When we get to El Pilar, you will see exactly how the cacao is handled. Then you two will be experts!" Jesús laughed and we laughed, all of us knowing that only a career dedicated to cacao can really yield all the subtle secrets of the plant. But we were happy to have an insider's view and to take in the sights, sounds, smells, and flavors of cacao.

Pulling up to the gates of the 625-acre Agropecuaria plantation, we were greeted by Carlos, an energetic farm manager, machete in hand. With his free hand, Carlos pumped ours with a grin before turning on his heels and setting a brisk pace into a vast, shady expanse of green cacao trees. As we followed along, we saw workers with long-handled steel blades cutting ripe cacao fruits from trees. Jesús commented, "The very first part of our harvest work is the *recolección*, the actual cutting of the fruits from the trees. You have to be very careful to cut the fruit clean from the tree without damaging the tree in any way. This of course is no problem for a skilled cutter. Our men can harvest ripe cacao very quickly without damage because they have a lot of experience."

At Agropecuaria, the harvest period lasts about 5 months. During that time, cacao fruits ripen according to their own biological schedules, so fruits on the same tree may be harvested months apart from one another. The cutters in the plantation go through the trees over and over until all healthy ripe fruits are harvested. As we made our way deep into the plantation, we saw many men cutting cacao fruits and placing them in large baskets.

In a clearing, several men sat on logs, machetes in hand, cutting cacao pods and scooping out the insides with their blades. The fruits of their labors lay piled high in a colorful heap of red and yellow and white. Carlos explained, "After the men have cut the fruit, then comes the *partida y desgranada*, the separating of the beans from the fruit. The men cut the fruits open with a machete and then they scoop out the beans and the white flesh around them. So then you have this big pile of fruit, all cut open." The men kept a steady rhythm going, deftly cutting and scooping out one cacao pod after another.

We headed still deeper into the plantation, treading soft, warm ground between cacao trees whose leaves glistened in the sweltering tropical sun.

Hot, Sticky Beans

Approaching a large barn, Craig and I remarked at the sweet, floral, delicious chocolate aroma wafting in the hot air. "It's like chocolate and a sweet vinegar," Craig noted. As we entered the barn, the atmosphere was thick with the pungent, humid scent of fermenting cacao. Inside, we found several rows of large wooden bins; every other one was filled with gooey-looking cocoa beans. In a couple of bins, workers stood knee high in rubber boots, shoveling fermented beans from one bin to the next. "That way the beans that were on the top before are on the bottom. This results in more even fermentation," Carlos said.

Jesús explained the whole process. "After the cacao fruits are cut open and the beans are separated, the beans undergo *fermentación*, where they are put into these big wooden bins in the barn, and they ferment. All of the soft, fleshy fruit around the beans dissolves. That is where you get the most changes in the bean." During fermentation, the naturally purplish beans become brown, and the temperature inside the vat reaches 125 degrees Fahrenheit. The germ inside is killed, and enzymatic activity forms compounds that produce the characteristic cocoa flavor when the beans are eventually roasted.

Craig and I sniffed closely at the beans. "Go ahead," encouraged Jesús. "Stick your hands right down in there." Craig raised an eyebrow and shot me a sidelong glance. I shrugged. After rolling up a shirtsleeve, I plunged my arm up to the elbow into a vat of warm, sticky, fermenting cocoa beans. Craig did the same. It felt like I had sunk my arm into a pot of cooking baked beans.

"It's pretty hot in there, alright," I remarked to Jesús. He nodded affirmatively with a satisfied smile, evidently pleased that we were seeing every aspect of Agropecuaria San José, including the barn of fermenting vats. When I withdrew my arm from the beans, it made a sucking sound. My arm was mottled with sweet, viscous goo. "You have a hose?"

From the fermentation barn, Carlos and Jesús led us to an area where cocoa beans dried in rows on a series of large, elevated concrete platforms about waist high. A man in a wide-brimmed straw hat used a flat, long-handled shovel to turn the beans. Even going at a slow pace, the turning of the beans was hard labor in the broiling sun. The heat on the beans filled the air with the smell of warm cocoa. Carlos gestured with his machete as he told us about drying. "After the beans are fermented, then you must dry them. This *secado* takes place on a flat surface. You will see on the roads around here, the small cacao growers will dry their beans on the sidewalk, or even on the road. But we have many tons to dry, so we have these platforms. We must get the beans down to 8 percent moisture, so they will not spoil. They will lose almost half their weight. The beans will dry for a few days." Considering that the at-

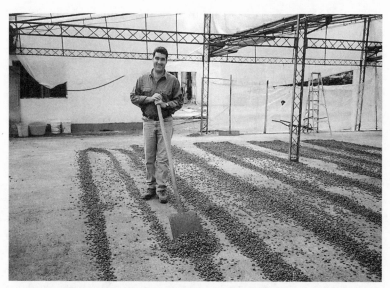

K. C. Miller of Chocolates El Rey turns cocoa beans as they dry.

mospheric humidity was 75 percent, the drying of the cocoa beans was a battle between heat and water.

Jesús picked up where Carlos left off. "After the drying is *limpieza*, the cleaning of the beans to remove any debris. But you will see that even as the beans are drying, many of the broken pieces and foreign materials will be picked out. Then when the beans are well cleaned, the last step is *clasificación*, where the beans are sorted and graded according to three different sizes. Then the beans are put into sacks, and they are sold to chocolate producers" such as El Rey and other manufacturers. He held a finger in the air to emphasize a point. "We get the cocoa beans ready. But the chocolate makers— they are the artists. They use these beans to make beautiful chocolate." Jesús broke into a big smile and closed his eyes, as if reflecting upon some special sweetness.

Chocolate Alchemy

Timothy Moley possesses the intensity of a man who has seen a grand vision of other worlds and won't be satisfied until you believe him. An ardent proclaimer and promoter of chocolate, Moley is the creative and discerning force behind the highly distinguished Chocolove brand. He started working in the spice industry as a teenager right out of high school, and that trade, with its exotic tastes and aromas, set him on the path that eventually delivered him to chocolate. During his time in spices, Moley traveled the world twice. This peripatetic touring exposed him to a world of flavors. "I tasted cuisine from 25 different countries, where people have incorporated a whole host of flavors. It had a huge impact on me."

After his spice travels, Moley worked in the herbal tea industry, where he played a key role in flavor blending. He also lived for a couple of years in the heart of California wine country, where he sampled the very best of that region's vintages. These many years of experience all came to bear on his career in chocolate. "When I set out to determine which product was a natural extension of my personality, chocolate was a perfect selection."

Moley's first efforts as a chocolatier were private ones, and initially he entertained no notions of hoisting the food of the gods onto his shoulders and helping to carry it forward into popular culture. "At first I began making chocolates for friends. They enjoyed it very much, and that pretty much sealed it. They kept saying to me, 'Make some more,' and so I did." As he spent more time in the kitchen slowly simmering chocolate at low heat, Moley became possessed by the bean and its sensuous, flavorful secrets. "For me, I enjoy chocolate on many levels. I enjoy the texture, I enjoy the complexity. Every batch is different. I enjoy the play of the flavors as they come out of the chocolate. It's a natural attraction for me. I like chocolate, and I like how I feel when I eat chocolate. Chocolate makes me feel pleasantly alert. I get stimulated and calm at the same time. My guess is that when early peoples consumed chocolate, they felt a heightened sense of awareness. Here was something exterior to the body that they could use to improve their performance, mentally and physically. For me, the chocolate experience is big. It affects people on a number of different levels all at once. I get a great deal of joy from chocolate, and I want to share that joy with other people."

Captivated and completely charmed by chocolate's reverie, Timothy Moley made chocolate his life path. "When I surveyed the U.S. market, it became clear to me that there was nobody in this country making a premium chocolate bar." And that is precisely what Moley set out to do. Bringing to bear his many years of flavor experience and his natural inclination toward perfection, he began to sample chocolates from all over the world. Blending one type with another, he tried numerous combinations of chocolate until he settled on a proprietary mix of African and Caribbean cocoa beans. Today, Moley's Chocolove brand comes in various strengths, including the 70 percent cocoa content Strong Dark version, which is the brand's signature bar.

To further the notion that chocolate enhances feelings of love, Moley embosses a heart onto the label of each bar and includes a love poem inside each wrapper. His approach to chocolate may be creatively distinctive, but the way chocolate roped him in was not. Many is the chocolatier who has first tasted, then dabbled with, then became wholeheartedly devoted to chocolate. Many is the flavor artist who winds up spending countless hundreds of hours engaged in the finicky craft of producing just the right bonbon recipe, the perfect *sauce au chocolat*, the quintessential truffle. Chocolate is like a kohl-eyed harem dancer, sinewy in movement, graceful and coy. When chocolate turns its full charms on a prospective servant, they are not likely to slip away.

The cocoa drink, or chocolate, has an additional quality not shared by tea or coffee. Whereas the latter two retard metabolism and beneficially stimulate the nervous system if taken moderately, chocolate directly nourishes.

—Baron Ernst von Bibra, 19th-century botanist

It may surprise some readers to learn that chocolate can vary as widely in flavor and aroma as do wines. While many of the large commercial chocolate makers bang out commodity chocolate by the tons, with a consistent flavor profile aimed squarely at the Big Mac eater, there are others, including brands like Chocolove, El Rey, and Valrhona that apply the kind of attention to flavor that a fine chef puts into a delicate and well-seasoned sauce. These are not chocolates you cram into your mouth as you run for a train. These are chocolates to linger over. Like the harem dancer, they fix your attention. Like brilliant music, they tantalize you. Like a well-crafted mystery, they draw you in. Like floral scents wafting on a warm breeze, they tease your finer senses. Like ecstatic sex on crisp linens on a sunny spring day, fine chocolates make you want more.

Once dried cocoa beans reach the chocolate manufacturer, they continue the odyssey that commenced at harvest. The beans are further cleaned through special strainers called riddles, to remove any remaining debris such as small stones, bits of wood, and sack fiber. Now they are ready for roasting. It is universally acknowledged that the roasting process holds the secret to making beautiful chocolate, much the way that the ideal roast will bring forth the full flavor of coffee. Traditionally, cocoa beans were roasted on wide iron pans over open fires. But in modern chocolate manufacturing, roasting is performed in large, electrically powered machines. Commodity cocoa is typically roasted at between 248 and 266 degrees Fahrenheit. But finer cocoa intended for high-quality chocolate is roasted below 248 degrees. Today's computer-controlled roasting machines enable chocolate makers to achieve exactly the right color and moisture content.

After roasting, cocoa beans are cooled. They are then flowed through cracking machines that break their brittle outer shells. Forced between rollers, the beans are cracked, and the shells are separated by strong currents of air. The remaining inner bean pieces are known as the nibs. It is this precious material that is transformed into chocolate.

Once the cocoa shells and nibs are separated, the nibs are finely ground into cocoa paste. The pressure of the grinding rollers heats and liquefies the cocoa butter, which makes up 50 percent of the volume of the nibs. This fatty liquid, rich with the fine starches and protein particles of the cocoa, is known as chocolate liquor. This liquor is allowed to cool and become solid.

The next step of chocolate making involves separating the cocoa butter from the solids. To accomplish this, the chocolate liquor is heated. Then it is put through a press. Most of the fine fatty cocoa butter goes one way, and the cocoa solids go another. The cocoa butter still contains some solids, and so it is filtered until it is pure fat. The pale yellow cocoa butter is molded into large blocks that can be stored almost indefinitely. The cocoa solids, which still contain between 10 and 20 percent cocoa butter, are pressed into cakes that are as hard as a rock.

I am always amazed by the extraordinary extent of human ingenuity when I learn about processing methods such as those required to make chocolate. We toy and tinker and noodle and play and work with plant materials until we achieve a form of preparation that satisfies us. We do this with chocolate, sugar, wines, cotton, wood, and myriad other plants. The extent to which we throw ourselves into the preparation of plant products and the gigantic nature of the various plant-processing industries clearly demonstrates the extent to which we and plants are bound together. They influence us, we influence them, and the cycle never ends. We are bound by nature through-out all time.

The beverage of the gods was Ambrosia; that of man is choco-late. Both increase the length of life in a prodigious manner.
—**Louis Lewin, M.D.,** *Phantastica*

After the cocoa butter and solids have been separated, the cocoa-solid cakes are made into cocoa powder. The addition of potassium carbonate, known as the alkalizing process, in-creases the pH value of the cocoa, neutralizing the acidity. This changes the way the cocoa solids react with liquids. Non-alkalized cocoa powder will sit in a clump on the surface of water or milk. Alkalized cocoa powder will mix into the liquid in a suspension.

Couverture is the industry name for the material we know as chocolate. The ingredients of chocolate are cocoa solids, cocoa butter, sugar, lecithin, and vanilla. The cocoa solids are loaded into huge grinding machines, where they are ground into a very fine paste. To this paste, cocoa butter is reintro-duced. The amount of added butter will vary, depending on the type of chocolate being produced. Milk chocolate, which contains only 25 percent cocoa content, will contain milk solids and milk fat in addition to the other ingredients previ-ously listed. Strong, dark, 70 percent semisweet chocolate will contain less cocoa butter and less sugar than other chocolates.

When all the ingredients are mixed together, they un-dergo conching. This is when all the ingredients in the chocolate recipe are blended together until a totally smooth, creamy, homogeneous mixture results. Commercial conching machines can blend up to 5 tons of material at a time, a process that typically takes about 10 hours.

In the final stage of chocolate manufacturing, the liquid material is cooled in stages to approximately 82 degrees Fahrenheit and then gently heated to 89 degrees. This process, known as tempering, stabilizes the fat crystals in the chocolate. Tempering gives chocolate its characteristic sheen and texture. Once tempered, the chocolate is poured and allowed to cool. Thus, after a multitude of practiced steps, beginning with the cutting of ripe cacao from a tropical tree, we have at long last that exquisite delight about which people rhapsodize. By wizardly alchemical means, the food of the gods is ready for our pleasure.

Cacao History

Sometime around 1000 B.C., the Maya—whose civilization flourished from the Yucatán Peninsula to the Pacific coast of Guatemala—are believed to have cultivated the cacao tree for the very first time. According to legend, cacao cultivation was initiated by the third Mayan king, Hunahpu. The Maya so highly valued cacao that they used cocoa beans as currency.

The intrepid seafaring legend Christopher Columbus was actually the first nonnative to see cacao. In 1502, Columbus was aboard the *Santa Maria*, moored off the island of Guanaja on the coast of Honduras, when he was visited by an Aztec chief in splendid raiment bearing gifts. Among the cloth, copper objects, and wooden weapons presented to Columbus were cocoa beans, which neither he nor his crew recognized. The Aztec made a beverage of the beans for Columbus, who found it bitter. The Aztec called the drink *cacahuatl*. Though Columbus reputedly brought some beans back to the Spanish royal court along with numerous other treasures, they received only cursory attention. The real discovery of the value of cacao was left to a subsequent explorer.

In 1519, Hernán Cortés landed at Tabasco on Mexico's Gulf of Campeche. He and his crew marched on the Aztec capital of Tenochtitlán, where they were greeted by the Aztec ruler Montezuma. Mistaking Cortés for the legendary king-turned-deity Quetzalcoatl, Montezuma presented Cortés with a large load of cocoa beans from a vast cacao plantation. Unlike Columbus, Cortés quickly ascertained the value of the bean. The Aztec made a drink of finely ground cocoa beans mixed in water and beaten to a froth with a wooden stirring instrument called a molinet. The beverage was not at that time, in that culture, for common folk. Instead, it was the potation of the privileged. People of high rank, including members of the royal house, nobility, and warriors, drank cacahuatl. The great emperor Montezuma is said to have consumed as many as 50 goblets of the drink daily, including a large goblet before visiting his harem. Montezuma was a fortunate man. He had his choice of the finest chocolate in the realm and the company of the finest and fairest maidens as well.

When Cortés returned to Spain from the New World in 1528, he told of a widely consumed food made from the fruit seeds of a tree. Cortés and his *conquistadores* described great plantations of *Theobroma cacao* throughout Mexico. He reported, "On the lands of one farm, 2,000 trees have been planted; the fruits are similar to almonds and are sold in a powdered state." In Cortés, chocolate found the perfect proclaimer. His account of chocolate, its popularity and value, greatly piqued the interest of the Spanish. Cortés was chocolate's first and most important transcontinental messenger.

In 1544, a delegation of Mayan nobles visited the court of

Spain's Prince Philip. Among the many treasures they bore were cocoa beans. In 1585, the first commercial shipment of cocoa beans arrived in Seville with Spanish sailors returning from Veracruz. With a mighty and triumphant shout, cocoa crossed the great Atlantic Ocean. Its campaign to capture the palates of Europeans had begun in earnest.

The Europeans introduced a seminal element to the prized Aztec drink that would change the face of chocolate forever. Sugar was added to sweeten the bitter beverage, making it immediately pleasing to the European palate. Unlike the Aztecs, Spaniards drank their chocolate hot, not cold. Consumed as a sweet, hot beverage, chocolate became a symbol of status in the court at Madrid. From there, chocolate strode like a finely attired dandy into Spanish high society, where it was received with warmth and enthusiasm. Realizing the great commercial value of this delightful drink, the Spanish established cacao plantations in their overseas colonies. Great fortune, they realized, lay in pleasure.

I bring to you a special drink from far across the West,
Although it's nearest loves on whom it's said to work the best.
Good cheer it always brings, and your full years renews.
First take a sip, my dear, and I shall presently;
And know I serve it to you with all the warmth that's due:
For we must take good care to leave descendants for posterity."
—a late 18th-century love poem

Though Mexico was the original source of commercial cacao, the Spaniards discovered large forests of wild forastero cacao in the Guayaquil coast of Ecuador. By clearing other vegetation away from the cacao trees, the Spanish had a fast and easy source of cacao fruit, made even cheaper by slave labor. Compared with Mexico's fine criollo cocoa beans, the Ecuadorian forastero beans were less flavorful but more prolific. The Jesuits, too, found large stands of wild forastero cacao growing along the banks of the Amazon and its tributaries. And so it came to pass that cocoa beans from Mesoamerica and South America made their way by various means to an increasingly chocolate-hungry Europe.

Chocolate encountered a religious hurdle in 1591 when the question arose as to whether the consumption of the beverage broke the Lenten fast. The Jesuits, who traded in chocolate, contended that the ambrosial drink most certainly did not break the fast. By contrast, the Dominicans took up an opposing view. Eventually the issue came to Pope Gregory XIII, who declared that drinking chocolate did not break the Lenten fast. Score one for the Jesuits and for chocolate. Just as with coffee, chocolate advanced with papal approval.

Chocolate took handy advantage of the institution of matrimony with the 1615 marriage of Hapsburg-Spanish princess Anna of Austria to France's Louis XIII. As one of many wedding gifts, Anna presented a casket of chocolate to Louis. The pampered princess also brought with her a maid to prepare her daily chocolate. By virtue of this fortuitous conjugation, chocolate slipped across family lines and international borders to become the favored drink of the French court.

A short while later, chocolate made its way from France to Italy. The sweet, sensuous flavor and feel of the beverage appealed greatly to the Italians, whose sensibilities of luxury were similar to those of the Spanish. Chocolate fit the romance-language nations like a soft hand in a tailored velvet glove. The drink of cocoa, sugar, cinnamon, vanilla, and water soon became a staple.

In the 17th and 18th centuries, neither Mexico nor Ecuador was the primary supplier of cocoa beans to Europe. Instead, Venezuela, with its highly prized Caracas criollo, was number one. Spanish and Dutch traders sailed ships laden with Venezuelan criollo to eager European markets. At the same time, the scenic West Indies became home to sprawling cacao plantations. Martinique, Guadalupe, Jamaica, Hispaniola, and Trinidad all became important suppliers of cocoa beans. In Trinidad, the cross-pollination of criollo and forastero varieties led to the development of trinitario cacao.

Continuing its steady move around the world, chocolate sailed the short distance across the English Channel, and in 1657 the first of many English chocolate houses opened on Bishopsgate Street in London, quickly followed by numerous others. Among the most notable were the Cocoa Tree and White's. Much later, in 1824, Quaker John Cadbury opened a coffee and tea shop in Birmingham, where he also sold hot chocolate. Cadbury would become one of the world's great chocolate dynasties.

The invention of a mechanical, steam-driven chocolate grinder in 1700 changed the fundamentals of the chocolate industry. A labor-intensive process performed by hand in small quantities became a matter of mass production. As a result of the sharp reduction in labor costs, chocolate prices tumbled and the drink became economically accessible to the average person. The 19th-century botanist Baron Ernst von Bibra explained the then-popular process of preparing a liquid dose of chocolate, as opposed to the solid form we so often reach for today:

> Chocolate of fine and good quality is prepared by crushing the roasted and husked beans between rollers, then mixing them with sugar, vanilla, or occasionally with other spices, and allowing this mixture to cool. The chocolate beverage is prepared in various ways: it is simply boiled with water, with some sugar added to it. But it is also consumed with the unavoidable milk, with a lot of sugar, or with eggs. Since chocolate is actually a thin paste or soup, and its infusion is not prepared from cacao seeds or leaves as in the case of tea or coffee, it is more appropriate for chocolate than for the two other beverages to be taken with toast, cookies, and all kinds of other things.

In 1819, Francois-Louis Cailler built the first Swiss chocolate factory in Corsier, near Vevey. The Swiss would further advance chocolate's fortunes with innovation. In 1875, Vevey-based partners Daniel Peter and Henri Nestlé turned out the world's first milk chocolate. The Swiss enjoyed exclusive manufacturing of milk chocolate until the British firm Cadbury developed its process for the same product in 1904. But it was Rudolph Lindt who discovered perhaps the greatest secret of chocolate making—conching. As a result of mixing chocolate for several days and adding more cocoa butter, the confection melted in the mouth. This transformed chocolate manufacturing everywhere, and today all manufactured chocolate is conched.

In 1889, Jean Tobler, a former confectionery trader, founded the Tobler factory in Berne, Switzerland, with his sons. Their famous Toblerone bar was made in the shape of the Swiss Alps and contained chocolate with a nougat of almonds and honey. And in 1907, the Perugina chocolate factory was founded by Giovanni Buitoni and family. Playing up the love connection, Perugina made the first chocolate "kisses" by wrapping their bonbons in love missives.

It was a prescient event when cocoa beans from the West Indies landed in Dorchester, Massachusetts, where John Hanan established the first North American chocolate factory. Before long, two U.S.-based companies would become titans in the world of cacao. Hershey's Chocolate was founded in 1895 by Milton Hershey, and archrival Mars Incorporated was founded by Frank Mars in 1922. Both companies would in time generate not only mountains of chocolate products, but staggering wealth as well.

Today, chocolate is consumed widely throughout Europe and the Americas, and to a lesser extent in other parts of the world. Large commercial cacao plantations operate in Brazil, Cameroon, Colombia, the Dominican Republic, Ecuador, Ghana, Indonesia, the Ivory Coast, Malaysia, Mexico, Nigeria, and Papua New Guinea. Smaller plantations can be found in just about every other tropical location. Chocolate, the food of the gods and the electuary of lovers, has come to captivate humanity. Well done, chocolate. Bravo! The world would be a poorer place without you, the preferred pleasure of children and poets alike.

The Marvelous Methylxanthines

As I have previously mentioned, chocolate is a veritable cornucopia of naturally occurring compounds. Of this multitude, the most comprehensively studied are the methylxanthines. The two methylxanthines found in chocolate are caffeine and theobromine. Compared with coffee, chocolate is a poor caffeine source. According to the Chocolate Information Center, a 50-gram piece of dark chocolate—about the size of your average chocolate bar—will yield between 10 and 60 milligrams of caffeine, while an average 5-ounce cup of coffee can yield up to 175 milligrams. Nonetheless, chocolate can give a mild caffeine lift.

Theobromine, the other methylxanthine in chocolate, occurs at a concentration of about 250 milligrams in a 50-gram bar of dark chocolate. Like caffeine, theobromine stimulates the central nervous system, although it is appreciably weaker. Theobromine is, however, a stronger cardiac stimulant and a more potent diuretic. Because this compound has a different chemical structure than caffeine, we can assume that it possesses its own unique effects, but at present these effects are not yet well researched.

The presence of both caffeine and theobromine certainly contribute to the overall mood-modifying effect of chocolate, even if it is not an especially potent stimulant per se. Rather, chocolate is a complex cocktail whose multitudinous compounds come at the brain in a thousand ways, creating a delightful and unique reverie that no other substance can replicate.

Chocolate and Your Heart

All too often, we learn in the news that something we enjoy is bad for us. In a wonderful twist of fortune, we have discovered quite the opposite with chocolate. Substantive science now shows that chocolate, that ardently adored confection for which there is no viable substitute, is very good for us indeed. According to a report in an issue of the *American Journal of*

Clinical Nutrition, chocolate is good for your heart. Cocoa, which is the primary ingredient in finished chocolate, is rich in antioxidant polyphenols, a group of protective chemicals found in many plant-based foods and beverages such as red wine and tea. These have been the focus of scientific investigation for their beneficial influence on cardiovascular health.

Polyphenols are reportedly cardioprotective in two ways. First, they help to reduce the oxidation of low-density lipoproteins (LDL), or so-called bad cholesterol. Oxidation of LDL is considered a major factor in the promotion of coronary disease, most notably heart attack and stroke. Additionally, polyphenols inhibit blood platelets from clumping together. This clumping process, called aggregation, leads to atherosclerosis, or hardening of the arteries. By inhibiting aggregation, polyphenols reduce the risk of atherosclerosis. Since atherosclerosis is a major killer of American adults, the protection provided by the polyphenols in cocoa is of real value.

According to work conducted at the Department of Nutrition at the University of California, Davis, cocoa not only inhibits platelet aggregation, it also thins the blood, thus slowing coagulation. In a study of healthy subjects given a strong cocoa beverage, platelet aggregation was reduced and fewer microparticles than normal had formed. Additionally, blood took longer to form a clot than blood from control subjects. This study shows that cocoa performs the same beneficial anticlotting activity as aspirin. I'd rather drink a nice cup of hot cocoa any day than swallow baby aspirin to protect my heart.

UC-Davis researcher Carl Keen, Ph.D., noted in a study printed in the *American Journal of Clinical Nutrition* that the enriched flavonoid composition of the cocoa used in the study (less than the amount in two average cups of hot cocoa) may have contributed to the suppression of platelet activity after it was drunk. This work supports not only the concept that habitual cocoa consumption may be associated with improved heart health, but also that some positive effects may arise after the occasional cup. Dr. Keen adds, "Cocoa, and presumably other forms of chocolate, can be part of a healthy diet."

Before you go crazy and run down to the candy store to stuff your pockets with chocolate bars for your new cardiovascular enhancement program, though, there are a few facts to keep in mind. The UC-Davis work shows that the protective agents in chocolate are found in cocoa. Thus, the two very best ways to benefit from the heart-enhancing effects of chocolate are to either consume cocoa powder or eat a moderate amount of semisweet dark chocolate. Cocoa powder can be used liberally to make hot cocoa, using either milk (skim, if you are on a fat-restricted diet) or water, or it can be added to blender drinks and baked goods. You can also make a great mole sauce and enjoy your cocoa that way. Cocoa powder contains little fat and no sugar. Sweeten lightly to keep the sugar content down.

Semisweet dark chocolate will give you the highest amount of cocoa solids in a bar, with the lowest percentage of fat and sugar. For while cocoa in chocolate is highly healthful, there are well-established disadvantages to fat and sugar. If you are going to make chocolate your cardio supplement, then look for those brands, such as El Rey, Chocolove, or Valrhona, that offer bars containing 70 percent cocoa. Half a 90-gram bar will contain about 125 fat calories and more than 30 grams of cocoa. Now, I'm not saying to toss your heart medication in the trash, but this kind of natural heart protection is way more pleasurable and far less expensive than consuming a potentially dangerous cardiac drug. Plus, real semisweet dark chocolate offers the biggest fix of authentic chocolate flavor. Once you adjust to the rich and complex taste, you'll never go back to lesser chocolate.

What About All the Bad Stuff?

Everybody knows that chocolate causes acne, cavities, and headaches, right? In fact, these claims appear to lack any real substantiation.

Acne occurs largely as a result of either poor skin hygiene or changes in hormones. Assuming that the average chocolate eater washes his face and performs basic hygienic functions, what could account for the claim that chocolate causes acne? The answer seems to be that women as a group consume the most chocolate, and more so during menstruation (and hormonal fluctuations) than at other times. A woman menstruates, eats chocolate, gets pimples, and makes a connection between the chocolate and the zits. But studies of individuals who consume large amounts of chocolate, including research conducted at the U.S. Naval Academy, show no evidence that chocolate causes or exacerbates acne. A lot of chocolate may make you fat, but at present there is no evidence to show that it will blemish your skin.

As concerns dental caries (cavities), the news about chocolate is glowingly good. Research shows that tannins in chocolate actually inhibit the production of cavities. That's right—chocolate actually helps to prevent cavities. This does not mean that you should skip brushing your teeth and eat chocolate instead before going to bed. But it does mean that you need not fret that consuming the food of the gods will bore holes in your teeth. For the record, raisins are the most cariogenic (cavity-causing) food known. They not only contain high amounts of sugar, but their sticky sugar lingers on the enamel of teeth, where it changes the pH of the surface, making it porous, thus promoting cavities. If you eat chocolate, don't worry too much about cavities. (And if you eat raisins, brush your teeth after doing so.)

The belief that chocolate causes migraines has resulted in research that has found no such connection. A study conducted at the University of Pittsburgh reported that "contrary to the commonly held belief of patients and physicians, chocolate does not appear to play a significant role in triggering headaches in typical migraine, tension type, or combined headache sufferers." Other studies have also found no connection. Now, if for some reason you get a whopper headache after eating chocolate, then don't eat it. But the research so far has failed to find any connection.

The Agony of Field Research

K.C., Craig, and I sat at a large conference table at the headquarters of Chocolates El Rey in Barquisimeto, Venezuela. Before us lay five plates piled high with different types of dark chocolate. K.C. poured from a bottle of chilled Venezuelan champagne into fluted glasses. "To cleanse the palate," he noted.

We were about to engage in organoleptic science, employing our highly refined sense organs of smell and taste to sample the chocolates before us, and to offer critical evaluation. We even had actual evaluation forms and pencils. After all, eating heaping piles of chocolate and washing it down with fine dry champagne is serious business. It requires dedicated professionalism and keen discernment. I knew to chew thoughtfully and sip slowly, to avoid coming off as a choco-late-chomping, champagne-swigging rube from north of the border.

"Okay, here's what we've got here," K.C. explained. "Each of these chocolates is a 70 percent cocoa chocolate, and each one is made from a different cacao from a different region." He explained that at Chocolates El Rey, they approach choco-lates like good wineries approach various vintages. Just as a Napa Valley winery might produce a cabernet sauvignon, so too Chocolates El Rey produces varietal chocolates from cacao harvested at specific plantations, with remarkable dif-ferences in flavor and aroma.

K.C. proceeded like a professor on the opening day of a science class. "This one is Macuro, from the Rio Caribe area. This one is Gran Saman, made from our special Carenero Su-perior cocoa beans from the Barlovento area, in north-central Venezuela. This one here is Apamaté, also a Carenero Supe-rior bean, but a different mix of cacao solids and cocoa butter. This one is Sur Del Lago from south of Lake Maracaibo, and this one, San Joaquin, is made from an Ocumaré bean from Barinas state. So what I recommend you do is take any kind, chew it slowly, and just let it melt in your mouth, so you can really taste the subtle flavors." Craig and I needed no further urging. We picked up pieces and began tasting.

It is a wonderful thing to spend a hot, sticky afternoon in South America sitting in a cool place tasting superb chocolates and drinking fine champagne. It is even more wondrous still to experience highly distinct differences between dark choco-lates. Each of the five chocolates was unique and excellent, and I wondered what the heck I had been eating all the years prior to that day. But two stood out above the rest. The Gran Saman possessed intricate earthy and woody flavor notes and finished with a soft, lingering bitterness. But the San Joaquin narrowly won the day, possessed of a complex sweetness and a lingering smokiness. K.C. laughed when Craig and I both announced the San Joaquin as a favorite. "You can't even get that one in the States. Every kilo we make goes right to Japan." He paused for effect. "Of course, I could send you home with a few kilos."

After we had chewed our way through all five varieties, we sat peaceful and happy, luxuriating in the pleasant mood that fine, dark chocolate provokes. The afternoon was heading toward dusk, and it was no time to throw ourselves into vigorous work. Rather, we relaxed and told stories and whiled away the time, under the subtle but lovely influence of the food of the gods.

Chiles
Hellfire in Your Mouth

They're known by various names: chiles, chilies, chilis, cayenne, and plain old hot peppers, among others. Interestingly, chiles were misnamed "peppers" by Christopher Columbus and his crew, who likened them to the pepper of India, *Piper nigrum*. Though chiles are not really a *Piper* at all, the name has stuck. Proper or not, chiles are peppers, and that's the way of things.

Whatever you call them, chiles are not demure vegetables that sit off in the corners of the mouth like the gentle flavors of eggplants and pole beans. The fiery chile demands even more notice than pungent garlic. Used as food, medicine, and even weapons, and as the main protagonist in trial-by-ordeal pepper-eating contests, chiles are the left-wing activists of the salad kingdom, the most intense, strident, take-charge veggies in the world.

A concatenation of cultural causes has created the climate in which the blistering chile burns inexorably toward absolute world immolation of the oral cavities of the masses. In other words, interest in hot, spicy foods has soared astronomically over the past couple of decades. In 1992, salsa sales exceeded ketchup sales in the United States. The implication of this fact is staggering. America has traded her favor of sweet and tangy table sauce for the licking flames of chile fever. An insatiable appetite for gustatory heat is blowing around the planet like a scorching sirocco. People just can't get enough of hot chiles, those firecracker flora of the genus *Capsicum*, whose heat levels range from moderate to thermonuclear.

The Dreaded Chac Mool

I was, as the oft-employed expression goes, minding my own business. I felt hungry as well, and this abdominal vacuity impelled me toward a small and rustic eatery called Chac Mool, in Playa del Carmen, on the eastern coast of Mexico's Yucatán Peninsula. The smell of food wafting through the slat walls was tantalizing. Inside, a dirt floor was packed hard from years of footsteps. A filthy, lazy fan stirred humid air inside the shack, and flies buzzed my head. I sat down carefully on a wobbly wooden chair whose joints were about to give out, at an equally shaky card table with cheap plastic cover.

I made two mistakes. First, I asked for the *comida del Dio*, which brought a sputtering, red-faced laugh from the waiter. I had asked for the food of God, which they apparently didn't serve. Stupid gringo. I duly noted the error and requested instead *comida del día*, the special of the day. In mere minutes, a plate of sizzling grouper, steaming rice, refried beans, and crispy fried plantain arrived at my table. A cold Modelo Negro beer and salsa accompanied, and I dug in like a miner picking at a rich gold vein. But the salsa, with its tomatoes and onions but no apparent chiles, conveyed not even a trace of heat. So I asked an innocent enough question: "Don't you have anything hotter?" That was the second mistake.

In retrospect, I should have registered the flicker in the waiter's eyes, the slight nod of the cook's head in the kitchen, the silent moment that passed between us all. But I was distracted by the happy sensations of hunger being satisfied, with absolutely no sense of impending doom. Not even when the waiter turned silently on his heel and headed briskly toward the kitchen. Not even when he returned equally silently, set down a small bowl before me, and said curtly, *"En-yoy."* I gave a questioning look at the bowl, which contained a fluid as clear and thin as water and what looked like two tiny orange nail parings at the bottom. As far as I could figure, the waiter hadn't understood my request. But just in case the liquid offered some flavor, I splashed it carelessly onto my food and dug in.

When the fire came on, it shot through me like a flaming Stinger missile. The cavity of my mouth was not big enough for the explosive fireball. My lips made a big, python-wide *O*, and I gasped in exclamation once before my throat closed off. As though I had swallowed lit gasoline, my throat seized and burned in anguish. Blood rushed from my neck to the surface of my face with such rapidity that I felt as though my skin would rip off in strips. My optic vessels strained and bulged, and I became furiously bug-eyed. My hands automatically gripped the sides of my skull, as though to prevent my parietal bones from blowing. Through blurry, bloodshot vision, I caught the waiter's eye. "Hot, yes?" he commented without expression. Hot, hell yes. Volcano hot. Flamethrower hot. The Great San Francisco Fire hot. Hotter than Dante's Inferno. Hotter than molten steel.

In a desperate act as a man aflame, even as my oral membranes were frying, I jammed a beer bottle into my mouth and jerked my head back. As the cool, carbonated beverage raced down my throat, I strained a panicked eye at the waiter and jabbed furiously toward the bottle with the index finger of my free right hand—the universal request for a second round, quickly please. He brought another speedily, and I downed that brew on the spot. But the burning did not stop nor diminish even a little. I quickly blew breath out rounded lips to cool my mouth. I even closed my eyes and tried to meditate away the pain. Forget about it. I just sat there, feeling the hellfire in my mouth, completely stoned from the chile heat.

Stoned? Yes, pleasantly stoned. You see, here's the secret of chiles. People don't eat superhot peppers because they like the sensation of mucous membranes being seared raw. No, chile aficionados like the evil little vegetables because they cause the brain to produce profuse amounts of endorphins, morphinelike substances that can alter your mental state significantly if you get enough going at once. The hot sauce I'd consumed was fiery enough to produce about a bucketful of endorphins. I was impressively high. And so, happily spaced on natural opiates, I sat on my rickety wooden chair and hung out until the excruciating heat in my mouth and throat subsided.

And then I proceeded as any true chile devotee would. I slowly and carefully finished my meal, bite by incendiary bite. Yes, my face was beet red and throbbing, and yes, tears streamed down my cheeks, and the blood in my ears pounded like giant Japanese ceremonial drums. But I was so whacked from the natural opiates bathing my brain that I truly enjoyed the pain. It was luscious. Ardent chile devotees are a sick bunch, though I make no apologies for being one. When I finished the meal, I reached into my shirt pocket, pulled out a bill, dropped it onto the table, and shambled woozily into the Yucatán sun with a stupid grin on my face. I dropped nearby on the ground in the shade of a coconut tree and fell into a swooning, deliriously high sleep for about an hour.

After the first mouthful, the tears started to come. I could not say a word and believed that I had hellfire in my mouth. However, one becomes accustomed to it after frequent bold victories.
  —Ignaz Pfefferkorn, 18th-century Jesuit missionary in Mexico

I suppose I should have paid more attention to the name of the eatery. Chac Mool was a god introduced to the Maya by the fierce warring Toltecs, who offered human sacrifices to the sun. A typical image of Chac Mool has him reclining, cradling a head in his lap. (Your Head on a Platter would have been another great name for the restaurant.) I also could have boned up a little on my chile lore before casually requesting something hotter. The Maya, whose brilliant culture flourished throughout the verdant Yucatán Peninsula and Guatemala, were not only master architects, builders, and astronomers, but they knew a few things about chiles too. And they had at their disposal one of the world's hottest varieties to play with.

To put the fiery habanero, the chile of the Maya, into perspective, consider the heat of the hottest jalapeño, at

5,000 Scoville Units—the universally recognized measure of chile heat (see "Scoville, Measurer of Fire" on page 112). Many is the person who has been surprised and burned by jalapeños. They are but child's play. The searing habanero pepper weighs in at 300,000 Scoville Units—a full 60 times hotter. The crafty Maya figured out how to marinate the skin and hot-oil-bearing seeds of the habanero in vinegar and lime juice to produce a clear liquid that is so blazing hot, it's like licking the surface of the sun.

The Legend of the Chile

Long ago, more than 10,000 cycles of the brilliant beaming sun ago, before the great cities of the Maya, the Aztec, and the Inca, red-skinned native peoples roamed the hills and forests of the great continent of South America. At that time, a hunter was stalking game deep in the dark green forest of what is now Bolivia, pursuing a large tapir with a wooden spear. The animal was elusive, but the hunter was expert. He knew to stop and be silent, to listen carefully, to move with the breeze, to stay downwind, and to remain patient.

As the hunter carefully stalked his way through the woods, he came upon a bush that he had never seen before. The bush grew as high as his chest and was abundantly laden with slender red fruits the length of his fingers. The hunter was curious. He touched the smooth, attractive fruits and admired their shiny skin. He wondered of their flavor. Were they sweet or sour? Picking one, he put the fruit to his mouth and took a bite. His eyes flew open with great surprise as the fruit produced a strong burning sensation in his mouth. What was this, some type of spirit medicine?

The hunter was cautious. He knew that many fruits and foods could be discovered in the forest and that one must approach each with care, to understand its secrets and appreciate its uses. Forgetting all about the tapir, the hunter collected a small satchel of the red fruits and hurriedly returned to his village many hills away. There, he presented the fruits to the curer, who knew many plants of the forest and understood how to treat many ills.

"Have you ever seen such a fruit before?" asked the hunter.

"No, in all my days I have not seen such a fruit as this," replied the curer as he turned over one of the fruits in his hand. He asked the hunter a number of questions about the location of the bush, the number of fruits, and what other plants grew nearby. Did the bush grow near running water? Did the hunter see any birds eating the fruits? Was there any evidence that animals partook of the fruits? What kinds of animal tracks were found nearby? Cautiously, the curer took a small bite of one fruit and chewed. The fruit was indeed potent! The curer sat quietly, allowing the heat in his mouth to gradually subside. He also noticed a pleasant feeling in his mind and body, a sense of peace and delight. He smiled with deep knowing. "This surely is a special fruit, a spirit fruit," he declared. "We must know this plant, which the spirits have placed in your way. This is good fortune." The curer directed the hunter to take him at once back into the woods to where the mysterious plant grew.

The two men returned to the plant. For a long time the curer carefully observed the bush, its branches and leaves, and the way the fruits hung and clustered. He knew many plants but had never seen nor heard of one such as this. He cut a branch laden with fruits and looked at it as though seeing within. He chanted and thought, and at last he spoke. "This is a sacred plant," he told the hunter. "We will take the seeds, and we will plant them in soil near our village. We will learn the nature of this plant, and it will bring us goodness." The curer and the hunter returned to the village where their relatives and friends gathered with interest and curiosity. "On this day we have been given a new gift from the spirits," declared the curer.

One of the women in the village was cooking game and roots in a pit, and she asked the curer for several of the fruits, which she pounded with a heavy piece of wood until they were well-mashed. She added the pounded fruits to the game and roots and covered the food with leaves. The food in the pit cooked overnight until tender, and the woman removed the covering leaves upon the rising of the morning sun. She served some of the food to the curer, the hunter, and other members of the village. At first, each was surprised by the heat of the new fruit. But they liked it! Somehow, the fruit made them laugh and feel light in their hearts. When one person expressed surprise by the sudden heat, the others would point and laugh. Some grew red in the face, some came to tears, yet still they smiled. The people sat together and enjoyed the hot food, remarking at the great good fortune that had been bestowed upon them by the spirits.

Chile Reverie

What divine secret lies at the sacred heart of the piquant chile? What deep mystery does it reveal? Does the mere zesty snap of chile in a good recipe alone account for why so many blister themselves for this vegetable? Or does a force more grand steer the appetites of the millions?

Beelzebub's favorite vegetable woos the faithful with a seductive religious experience of chapped and burning lips, a spanked and swollen tongue, a mouth that aches with heat, a searing swallow, a gastric churning, sweat drooling down a sizzling brow, face flushed with hot pounding blood, and a wave of pain-quenching endorphins that surge in the brain like firemen in a city aflame.

Chiles rage down the esophagus and into the GI tract, spreading fire deep into the belly, blowing steam out the ears of their most ardent devotees. In the blinding grip of chile fever, the mind swoons in ecstatic pain, like an acolyte with stigmata.

Chile reverie is a zealous devotion all its own. Hot-pepper pilgrims will travel far and wide for a hotter hot sauce, a fiery chile festival, a restaurant whose salsa is the stuff of burning legend. Why, oh why, do people subject themselves to this blazing ordeal? It's the pleasure, brain cells swimming in endorphins, being drunk and giddy on natural opiates, happy-faced and silly high.

Of all the psyche delicacies, only chiles occupy such a prominent place in food preparation. Chiles can be used in just about any kind of dish, from meat, fish, and vegetables to soups, stews, salads, and desserts. Name the food—how about orange juice or chocolate cookies?—and chile aficionados have found a way to insinuate the devil's vegetable into it.

Chiles offer one of nature's greatest highs. They are abundant. They are cheap. They are legal. They are the hottest thing.

The Plant

What is this mysterious plant whose pods yield fire and whose use has spread like licking flames through the culinary world? For our purposes, the chile plant is any of five domesticated species, including *Capsicum annuum*, *C. frutescens*, *C. pubescens*, *C. chinense*, and *C. baccatum*. These species are descendant from more than 20 wild species from tropical and subtropical America originally found in Bolivia, Mesoamerica, and Amazonia. All chiles may have originated from a single source, which some experts believe lies in central Bolivia.

Leave it to taxonomists to wrangle over the origins and genealogical lines of the chile plant; specifics matter little for our purposes. Suffice it to say that the chile is a cultivated perennial shrub as short as 12 inches and rarely taller than 7 feet in height, with profuse, asymmetrical light to dark green leaves and small white or purple flowers. The plant bears numerous fruits (chiles) of varying size, color, and heat. Of the domesticated capsicums, *C. annuum* is the most commercially significant and widely cultivated. Sweet bell peppers are included in this group, but since they lack any heat at all, they are of no concern to us here. They are wonderful vegetables, loaded with nutrients and beneficial antioxidant carotenoids, but they contain no fire, and I will not mention them again.

Though chiles originated in a hot, humid environment where they produced fruit year-round, the plant now thrives throughout temperate environments virtually anywhere there's a warm growing season. Thus, even in Canada, northern Europe, and the Himalayan foothills, chiles can be grown easily. Unlike their tropical cousins, however, they die at the onset of freezing temperatures, and like annuals they must be planted anew when warm weather returns. Almost any backyard garden can host a few chile plants. And if you peruse some of the more interesting seed catalogs such as Johnny's Selected Seeds or Nichols Garden Nursery, you will find uncommon varieties that grow well and easily, produce abundant fruits, and deliver enough fire to burn down the neighborhood.

This capsicum, or Indian pepper, is painstakingly grown in Castilia both by gardeners and by housewives. Instead of pepper it is used all the year round as a seasoning, either dried or in the form of the freshly picked green pods.

—Charles de l'Escluse, 16th-century cartographer

The fruits of the chile plant concern us most. Of these there is astonishing variety. Almost all chiles are green when immature, though some appear white or yellow or purplish. (I once encountered pale white chiles deep in the bush on southwest Espiritu Santo Island, in the South Pacific. They were screaming hot, and since the locals had no particular name for them, I dubbed them Santo Hots.) As a rule, mature chiles are red, orange, or yellow. This coloration is due to the presence of a red carotenoid known as capsanthin. The shape of chiles varies greatly. The cayenne variety is long, slender, and tapered; the cherry variety looks like a small tomato; the jalapeño is smooth and bulbous; the searing-hot chiltepin is small and shaped like a fat fingertip;

and the flaming habanero is bulbous and irregular. However, chiles do not conform to a specific size, shape, or
color, and there can be tremendous variations in heat level
among peppers of the very same species. One habanero may
be quite tolerable, but another may simply blow your head
off and leave you weeping and gasping for air. Chiles are
sneaky that way. You can never assume that you have them
figured out.

Chiles love nitrogen-rich soil, and they fruit most pro-
fusely when temperatures range between 70 and 80 degrees
Fahrenheit. Chiles require adequate moisture and cannot be
grown in dry soil. They grow best with regular rainfall or irrigation but drainage must be adequate. In those areas where
chiles are irrigated, they are often grown in raised beds so
the roots do not remain in water. According to some experts,
chile plants fruit more in geographic locations where the days
are shorter, between 8 and 12 hours of daylight, rather than
longer.

You might think that because of their pungency, chiles
would be poor targets for pests. But this is not the case.
Chiles are subject to infestation by cutworms, leaf miners,
weevils, aphids, and thrips. Chile shrubs can be attacked by
fungi, bacteria, various types of stem rot, and nematodes.
To counteract these various pests, large commercial farmers
employ a range of pesticides and herbicides. But truly savvy
growers employ organic methods, which build soil fertility
and increase resistance to pests and disease as a result of
vigorous plant health. Interestingly enough, since the advent of agrichemical use in the 1940s, the percentage of
crop loss due to pests has actually risen as the use of toxic
chemicals has increased. Add this to the fact that agrichem-
icals contribute to increased cancer rates among farm

workers while decimating wildlife and depleting the soil, and you have several compelling reasons to support organic agriculture.

Of the pepper I know little, except that it grows in very great abundance in the prairies west of the Sabine & that it is with the Spaniards and Savages, an article in as great use as common salt is among the inhabitants of the U.S.
—Thomas Jefferson, third president of the United States

Of the many places I have seen chiles under cultivation, the one that sticks in my mind most is outside of Bangalore, India. The farm, only a couple of acres in size, was tended by one peasant farmer and a helper. The chile shrubs were planted close together on raised beds, and the whole place was irrigated from a single standing, wide-mouthed pipe. The farmer was evidently dirt poor. He lived in a small mud hut without electricity or running water, his clothes were shabby and worn, and his glasses were cracked. He farmed without chemicals, and his hoe constituted the entirety of his weed-control program. He exuded a compelling warmth and pride, and he had much to be proud of. His chile shrubs glistened with robust vigor and were jam-packed with beautiful, pest-free fruits. His superabundant harvest of perfect chiles would ensure enough income to sustain his meager and fragile living.

I stood amidst the chest-high chile plants and took in the beautiful sight as a baking Indian sun beat down on us. I am always humbled by the noble work of farmers, without whom we could not eat. But I was especially impressed and struck by the sheer beauty of this man's chile farm. How hard farmers toil, with little recognition, under difficult conditions, battling weather and economics, with only modest remuneration, to produce such lovely foods that delight and please the palate. I picked off a small green chile and chewed it. Oh, it was plenty hot alright, and tears came to my eyes, but not because of the pungency of the chile.

Varieties

In the United States, the jalapeño and cayenne strains are the most widely grown of the chiles. Habaneros have become quite popular in recent years, but they still appeal primarily to heat freaks and not the general public. Most people who eat chiles simply want a little zip in their food, not a nuclear meltdown in the mouth. While chiles vary in heat, they also vary in flavor. Chefs and gourmands find their favorites, and the various chile sauces on the market today represent a stunning range of heat and taste.

As chile sauces proliferate, and as chile festivals and conventions become increasingly well attended, a wider variety of specialty chiles is being grown to fuel a fire-hungry market. More than 20,000 acres are dedicated to hot-pepper cultivation in the United States, while much larger acreage is dedicated in Mexico, India, and some other chile-producing nations. Beyond those that I've already mentioned, currently popular varieties of chile include carricillo, catarina, datil, de Arbol, fiesta, floral gem, fresno, Mirasol, NuMex, pasilla, penis (looks like a flaccid one), pepperoncini, rocotillo, rocoto, Santa Fe grande, scotch bonnet, serrano, tabasco, and Texan varieties. There are more, and my failure to mention them is not an intentional slight. Chiles are like apples, of which several dozen varieties are sold. You choose your favorites based on heat and flavor, and you find numerous ways to use and enjoy them.

Going to Extremes

The heat of the chile is measured in multiples of 100 units, from the bell pepper at zero Scoville Units to the incendiary habanero at 300,000 Scoville Units. That's hot! But even the hellish habanero has been surpassed by hotter peppers. The Mexican red savina variety of habanero has been tested at 575,000 Scoville Units. You would expect this extreme heat to secure a position for the red savina as the world's hottest pepper by a wide and uncomfortable margin. But another variety called the Francisca habanero is reputedly hotter than the red savina.

The Francisca may well have claimed the title of world's hottest pepper, but an even bigger scorcher has burst upon the chile scene. Specialists at Assam's Defense Research Laboratory in India reported in August 2000 that India's naga jolokia variety of *Capsicum frutescens* measures an astonishing 855,000 Scoville Units. Forget about it. That's just about hot enough to melt your teeth. Chile breeders, a hotly competitive bunch, are attempting to produce ever more fiery peppers. What is the point? Some chile aficionados simply want to be able to claim that they have survived consumption of the hottest peppers on Earth. I just have to shake my head and wonder, Will there ever be an end to the pain?

Harvesting

There are basically two ways to harvest chiles: by hand and by machine. For the most part, chiles are harvested by hand, and an average picker can harvest about 40 pounds of them per hour. In an 8-hour day, that comes out to about 320 pounds. Farmworkers are often paid by the amount of produce they harvest, so a picker who can bring in 400 pounds per day will make more money.

In the United States, commercial chile harvesting begins in mid-July and continues until all the chiles are in. Chiles do not ripen uniformly, so repeat picking is required. About every 7 days, farm workers go back through the fields and pick ripe chiles. A large farm can require several pickings.

More than 140 different mechanical harvesters have been devised to separate chile fruit from the plant. Commercial growers who employ mechanical harvesters grow chile shrubs that are uniform in size, typically short in height, and bear a lot of fruit to make it easier for these machines to harvest.

Curing

The majority of chiles undergo a curing process, except for those that are sold fresh in markets or are used immediately after harvest in commercial food manufacturing. Curing is basically a drying process and can be accomplished by several means. In the United States, Mexico, and other areas where chiles are grown on a large scale for commercial purposes, drying is usually accomplished in kilns or ovens that circulate hot air. The passage through the dryer on a conveyor belt can take as little as 15 hours or as much as 2½ days, depending on the type and size of the dryer. The most important thing is that the heat is consistent and the chiles are evenly dried.

Some types of chiles are dried in small or large quantities by smoking. These are usually thicker-fleshed varieties such as anchos and jalapeños. The chiles are placed in ovens in which drafts of air pull smoke from a fire beneath the chiles into a smoking compartment. When the chiles are fully smoked, they are called chipotles. Thus, when you see a salsa or a recipe that contains chipotle peppers, this refers not to a specific variety of chile but to those that have undergone the smoking process.

The most primitive method of drying involves ripening chiles on the shrub, turning off all irrigation, and allowing the chiles to wither until dry, prior to being picked. Other ways of drying chiles involve laying them out on mats, on concrete, on wooden floors, or roofs, and turning them regularly in the sun. In any and all cases, the curing of chiles reduces the fruits to one-fifth their fresh weight and results in a stable product that will keep for many years if stored in a dry place.

Hot Sauce

Great balls of fire! Have you looked at the names of chile sauces today? They give ample testimony to the extreme nature of the sauces themselves as well as that of their intended audience: Blair's Death Sauce, Mad Dog Inferno, Gib's Bottled Hell, Dave's Insanity, Acid Rain, The Final Answer, Brain Damage, Crazy Jerry's Mustard Gas, Scorned Woman, Widow, Screaming Sphincter, Endorphin Rush, Ring of Fire, Aspirin, Inner Beauty Real Hot, Bad Girls in Heat, Capital Punishment, Smack My Ass and Call Me Sally, and Pain Is Good. Is this not the sure decline of civilization as we know it? Lock your doors and keep your children away from these people.

Of course, that's impossible. Chiles are everywhere. Just look at the far and wide distribution of the world's most successful chile sauce, Tabasco Brand Pepper Sauce, made in

Avery Island, Louisiana, by the McIlhenny Company. It is not the hottest of hot sauces, though it is piquant enough. Still, there are very few places where you cannot find Tabasco Sauce. I have been served Tabasco Sauce in Lima, Peru; New Delhi, India; and Shanghai, China. I have enjoyed it on fish in Manaus, Brazil, and on pasta in Amsterdam; also in Tokyo, Toronto, London, Fiji, Vanuatu, Austria, Germany, and Italy.

We can thank the wild popularity of Tabasco Sauce for cracking the ketchup barrier and for spreading gustatory heat throughout all nations. Tabasco Sauce sits proudly on my kitchen counter in the large bottle and goes into almost every dish I cook. Tabasco Sauce rules. No kitchen is complete without it.

Trial by Fire

In London, the cuisine is like a perpetually foggy day—bland. This is changing slowly, as the clutches of the great empire slowly lose their grip upon the tongues of the masses. Indian food has always been the zesty, lively exception to the constipating British diet of white bread, bangers and mash, fish and chips, and cheese and head lettuce. In the Kensington district of London, there is a restaurant I patronize when in town called the Famous Kensington Tandoor. The place is not big, fancy, or, in fact, famous to any extent that I can tell, but the food is rock-solid good Indian.

One day, after a visit to the nearby Royal Geographic Society, I ducked into the Famous Kensington Tandoor for lunch. After perusing the menu briefly, I settled on a chicken vindaloo (a fiery curry) and a vegetable biryani (a rice dish) with some roti (round breads) and chai (spiced tea). A couple of minutes after I placed my order with the waiter, the maître d' approached my table. He wore a crisply pressed white shirt and conveyed the air of a gentleman. "Excuse me, sir. About your order . . ."

I knew what he was going to tell me and interrupted with a polite wave. "Yes, the vindaloo. I know it's hot. That's why I ordered it. No problem." He nodded without further comment and left.

I must look like somebody you want to scorch with hot chiles, or maybe I fit some sort of profile or seem too confident. Hell, I don't know. I like hot food; I never boast about it, and I don't go looking for trouble. Nonetheless, shortly after my brief exchange with the maître d', he returned with a small silver plate of long, slender green chiles. "Perhaps since you like hot food, you will enjoy these." He wagged his head and set the plate down in front of me. I leaned forward and looked to the kitchen, where two cooks stuck their heads out waiting to see what would happen next. All I wanted was lunch, and here I was with the whole staff wanting me immolated.

There was only one way to deal with the situation. I thanked the maître d' for being so thoughtful and selected the longest chile on the plate. Putting the whole chile in my mouth at once, I bit down on it, chewed it up without any change of expression, and picked up another. I held it in the air like a lollipop. The maître d' was plenty surprised, and he could not hide it. One of the cooks elbowed the other. I remained impassive, bit down on the second chile, and spoke with my mouth full. "Not bad." I nodded slightly with measured approval.

Sure, the chiles were hot. But I was damned if I was going to give ground. From that moment on, I was everybody's new friend. One of the cooks actually served me the vindaloo personally, and each of the wait staff asked me if I liked the food and would I come back. Chile lovers are a strange and per- verse bunch. First they want to burn you at the stake, then they want to be your friends.

The point of my story is that chiles have made their way even to the Kensington district of London, where plain food has been the rule for centuries. Chiles have arrived. Today, chiles are everywhere, from the sticky, gumbo saloons of the Louisiana Bayou to the jerk shacks of Jamaica, the markets of Madras, and the pepper gardens of Siam. Chiles and their sauces can be found almost everywhere on Earth, even in London. This is testimony to their seduction. Through their heat, through their endorphin-producing magic, they have won adherents, conquered continents, and changed cuisines.

Chilephiles and Chilephobes

While the ranks of chile devotees swell year after year, not everybody is an admirer. For some people, the same mecha- nism that produces pleasure in the chilephile produces pain and discomfort in the chilephobe, who genuinely dislikes chiles, finds the chile experience exquisitely uncomfortable, and wants no part of them.

For every pleasure—hot tub, massage, sex, a good cup of coffee, a glass of fine wine—there are those who derive none at all from it. Many factors account for this, including bio- individuality. Everyone is blessed with unique physiological nuances. Some people drink a small quantity of coffee and must be scraped off the ceiling for the shriekingly speedy feeling they get. Some people receive a foot massage and find the ex- perience wholly unpleasant. While this may be hard to believe for those of us who love these things, it is unquestionably true.

Chiles in History

The tale of chiles is one of jumping from plant to pot, one nation after another. As with the other psyche delicacies, chiles have leapt upon our backs, driving us onward with their pleasurable psychoactive properties, using us for transport and territorial conquest. Though we do not know exactly when chiles were first discovered, approximately 10,000 years ago appears to be a pretty safe bet. Chiles were among the very first crops cultivated in the Americas, sometime around 4000 B.C. Seeds found south of Mexico City date native chile use there to around 7000 B.C., while seeds found in northern Peru show chile use there around 2500 B.C. One thing is for sure: The use of chiles caught on and spread quickly along established trade routes throughout Central and South America and the West Indies.

Chile's historic spread throughout the markets and culinary traditions of the world was greatly aided by explorer Christopher Columbus, whom we all know sailed the ocean blue in 1492. On New Year's Day 1493, Columbus encountered chiles at the New World's first settlement, La Navidad, on what is now Haiti. Writing about *aji* (the native name for chile) in his journal, Columbus remarked that "the pepper which the local Indians used as spice is more abundant and more valuable than either black or melegueta pepper." In his journal writings from his second voyage to the New World, Columbus remarked, "In those islands there are also bushes like rose bushes which make a fruit as long as cinnamon full of small grains as biting as pepper; those Caribs and the Indians eat that fruit as we eat apples."

Fleet physician Diego Alvarez Chanca additionally commented on chiles, saying, "They use . . . a vegetable called aji, which they also employ to give a sharp taste to the fish and such birds as they can catch, of the infinite variety there are in this island [Haiti], dishes of which they prepare in different ways." When Columbus and crew returned to Spain from their second voyage to the New World, they brought peppers along with other plants and items of discovery.

In September 1493, Spanish court historian Pietro Martire d'Anghiera wrote about the New World on the basis of information imparted by members of the first Columbus voyage. In his *De Orbe Novo* ("On the New World"), he wrote,

> Something may be said about the pepper gathered in the islands and on the continent—but it is not pepper, though it has the same strength and the flavor, and is just as much esteemed. The natives call it axi, it grows taller than a poppy. When it is used there is no need of Caucasian pepper. The sweet pepper is called Boniatum, and the hot pepper is called Caribe, meaning sharp and strong; for the same reasons the cannibals are called Caribes because they are strong.

Though it may be hard to imagine today, the discovery of chiles was momentous. Europe was in the grip of pepper fever, and the tiny grains of black pepper (*Piper nigrum*) were so precious and sought after that they were dispensed singly and considered as valuable as currency. Prior to the introduction of spices from the Far East, European food was bland and by many accounts spoiled. Pepper and other spices such as cloves and cinnamon excited and awoke the European palate and covered the rank flavor and offensive aroma of bad food. Columbus and other sailors sought a quicker route to India, in part to obtain spices for an increasingly voracious European spice habit. The discovery of chiles, adaptable to a variety of climates and easy to cultivate, meant that the world had a piquant alternative to black pepper. Traders did not need to travel to India to load their ships with small grains of pepper. By bringing capsicum seeds to Africa and other parts of the world, they could plant the newfound pungent spice, trade it easily, and satisfy the palates of the Old World.

Portuguese traders, who had developed significant centers of commerce along the western coast of Africa in the 1400s, made their way to Brazil in 1500 and the West Indies in 1502. The Portuguese eagerly seized upon the commercial potential of New World crops such as maize, sugar, and chiles and spread them to Africa and India. A scant 40 years later, three different varieties of chiles were known and cultivated in India. From the African coast, traders made their way into the dark green heart of the African continent, where chiles became dietary fixtures. Though it was virtually inconceivable at the time, New World crops would change the eating habits of the Old World. The New World offered an astonishing cornucopia of agricultural products that could be grown in many other parts of the world. Corn, squash, coffee, chiles, cacao, tomatoes, avocados, lima beans, peanuts, potatoes, sweet potatoes, pineapples, vanilla, and manioc (cassava) would spread throughout the world and become staple foods. Tobacco, another New World plant, would also spread quickly, filling the lungs of the world with mildly narcotic smoke.

In the late 1520s, Spanish historian Bartolomé de Las Casas described three different varieties of aji found in the New World. Right around the same time, Portuguese sailors introduced chiles to Java. Eastern and Middle Eastern traders also carried chiles to New Guinea in the 1520s, and from there throughout Indonesia, Melanesia, and to Southeast Asia and China. Chiles became so integral to the cuisines of the East that they are thought to have originated there. In 1535, Spanish historian and navigator Gonzalo Fernández de Oviedo y Valdés chronicled the use of peppers in the southern

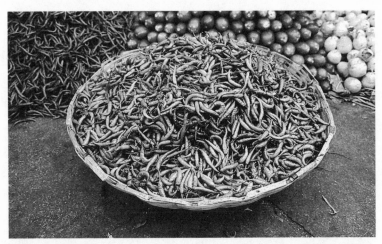

A large basket of chiles on display at Devaraja Market, Mysore, India.

Caribbean and commented that "the Indians everywhere grow it in gardens and farms with much diligence and attention because they eat it continuously with almost all of their food." Meanwhile, chiles were burning their way through Europe. By 1542, chiles were known and used in Spain, Italy, and Germany. At the same time that chiles were known in Goa in the mid-1500s, they had spread to the Balkans and Moravia. Today there is no memory of culinary traditions in India, China, and other parts of Southeast Asia that did not include chiles. What is Hunan cuisine without nasty dried red chiles to scorch the mouth? What would a Goan fish curry taste like without searing chile paste to burn the mouth and throat? One can only imagine.

Oddly enough, though chiles originated in the New World, they did not land on the shores of North America until 1621, when they were introduced to the eastern coast of Virginia by English traders who brought them from Bermuda. Chiles have had a place in North American cuisine since then, but not the major role that they have played in hotter climates. While chiles spread like roaring flames through dry timber between the Tropics of Capricorn and Cancer, they warmed up in North America more slowly. But since their victory over ketchup in 1992, they have burned hotter and brighter. Today, chiles are the bursting fireworks in our culinary New Year's celebration, the strident brass section in our gustatory Mardi Gras marching band.

The Blazing Capsaicinoids

The substances that make chiles hot, providing pleasure to chile aficionados everywhere, are natural capsaicinoids. These substances account for between 0.1 percent and 1 percent of the total composition of a chile pepper. Of these compounds, the hottest is capsaicin, which tips the scales at more than 16 million Scoville Units. Capsaicin was first discovered, isolated, and named in 1876 in India by an Englishman named L. T. Thresh. Pure capsaicin is a seriously dangerous material. A single drop of pure capsaicin will burn a hole right through healthy tissue.

Chemically, capsaicin is an acid. Capsaicin and dihydrocapsaicin together make up from 80 to 90 percent of the capsaicinoids found in peppers. The minor capsaicinoids include nordihydrocapsaicin, homodihydrocapsaicin, and homocapsaicin. The capsaicinoids open cell membranes in a way that allows calcium ions to flood into cells. This triggers a pain signal that is transmitted to the next cell. This is the same process that occurs when cells are exposed to excessive heat.

Because they are resinous compounds, the capsaicinoids are soluble in fats, oils, and alcohol. What this means to you is that in the event of a hot chile overdose, it does little good to pour water or any water-based substance like beer into your mouth to quell the fiery pain. In fact, doing so may actually aggravate your burning condition. A mouthful of cold water may close oral pores, sealing the blazing hot capsaicinoids inside. On the other hand, a swig of full-fat milk will liberate capsaicin from the pores in your mouth, thereby relieving your discomfort. In this case, milk acts as a surfactant, washing away fatty capsaicinoids in a manner similar to the way that soap washes away grease. Keep full-fat milk on hand for this emergency purpose. Forget skim, 1 percent, or 2 percent. You will perish in flames. Because alcohol is also an excellent solvent for the capsaicinoids, you can rinse your mouth out with a swig of tequila, vodka, grappa, or any high-octane liquor.

The capsaicinoids each possess a variation on what is known as a hydrocarbon tail. This tail enables the capsaicinoids to slip through lipid-rich cell membranes, producing a pervasive and persistent burning sensation. The slight structural variations in the hydrocarbon tail among the capsaicinoids changes their ability to penetrate layers of cells on the tongue, mouth, and throat. This structural difference may account for why some chiles burn in the mouth, while others burn deeper in the throat or stomach.

While chile peppers are mostly safe, high concentrations of capsaicinoids can be toxic and can actually destroy cells. For this reason, capsaicin makes an effective and highly painful weapon. The Maya burned chiles to incapacitate their enemies with blinding smoke screens, a nifty variation on tear gas. Their own insidious version of the grenade was a gourd filled with chile pepper extract. Today, capsaicin is the active ingredient in pepper sprays and is used by police to subdue dangerous individuals and by civilians to ward off muggers and dogs. The stuff is painful and dangerous. If you use a pepper spray, do so only in case of extreme emergency.

Scoville, Measurer of Fire

With more than a quarter of the world's population addicted to hot chiles, there's some hefty scientific research invested in the topic. One of the standards in the field is a well-articulated heat index, the Scoville Unit (SU) scale, by which all chiles are measured, from those chiles that are quite mild to others that are so blazing hot that they should not be eaten at all because they can burn right through the tough lining of the stomach.

In 1912, Wilbur Scoville, a chemist working for the Parke-Davis pharmaceutical company, established a method for measuring the heat level in chile peppers. In his original test, Scoville blended ground chiles with a sugar-water solution in increasingly diluted concentrations. A panel of testers then sipped the various dilutions, until they reached the point at which the liquid no longer produced a burning sensation. A number was assigned to each chile based on the extent to which it needed to be diluted before you could taste no heat. Thus, the Scoville Organoleptic Test was born.

Organoleptic is a term that refers to qualities that affect the senses. Organoleptic tests are widely used in the food, beverage, and fragrance industries to determine the quality of various products. Perfumery relies on olfactory organoleptic testing; the quality of coffees, wines, and teas is assessed by organoleptic taste tests; color testing for paint and wallpaper is a visual organoleptic test. Scoville's organoleptic test for chile peppers established a method for measuring their heat.

Though the accuracy of the Scoville Organoleptic Test has been questioned by some, chile heat is still always identified in Scoville Units. Today, though, the organoleptic testing procedure has been supplanted by a totally mechanical method employing high-performance liquid chromatography (HPLC). In this procedure, chile pods are dried, then ground. Next, they undergo a basic method of extraction, and the extract is analyzed. This method is appreciably more costly than tasting, but it measures the total heat of a pepper and also quantifies the amounts of the individual capsaicinoids present. By this sophisticated method, many samples can be analyzed within a short period.

As a result of all these tests, the varieties of chile peppers can be ranked according to their heat, or *pungency*, level. The following scale comes from research conducted by Dr. Ben Villalon of the Texas Agricultural Experiment Station. Dr. Villalon's findings have been reprinted and reproduced thousands of times; we in the chile world remain in his debt.

0–100 SU—bell/sweet peppers
500–1,000 SU—Big Jim, Anaheim
1,000–1,500 SU—ancho, pasilla
1,500–2,500 SU—sandia, cascabel, rocotillo
2,500–5,000 SU—jalapeño, Mirasol
5,000–15,000 SU—yellow wax, serrano
15,000–30,000 SU—de Arbol
30,000–50,000 SU—piquin, cayenne, tabasco
50,000–100,000 SU—chiltepin, Thai, santaka
100,000–300,000 SU—scotch bonnet, habanero
575,000 SU—red savina
855,000 SU—naga jolokia (do *not* try this pepper at home)
16 million SU—pure capsaicin (don't even think about it—ever)

A Duel, and a Burning Butt

In the summer of 1974, I found myself at a celebration of the summer solstice outside Española, New Mexico. The temperature registered in the 90s, and the utter lack of humidity gave the area the feel of Hell. Once again I was, as the saying goes, minding my own business. Some friends of mine knew that I enjoyed hot food, so they "kindly" introduced me to a man who claimed to share my passion for gustatory heat. Always glad to meet a kindred soul, no problem there. The man produced a handful of long, evil-looking, red de Arbol chiles and challenged me to eat one. The gauntlet had been thrown down. My friends crowded around, and I realized that the moment had been planned. That annoyed me enough to say I'd be happy to enjoy a chile, if my newfound acquaintance cared to join me. If I was going to go out in a ball of fire, I wanted some company. He frowned, caught in a trap of his own design.

With the groundwork for a chile-eating match thus established, we each picked a pepper. I smiled pleasantly, slipped the long, shiny red pepper into my mouth, and bit down. Damn, it was hot! Unreasonably, broilingly, heart-poundingly, blisteringly hot. But I was determined to keep my visible cool, even as my face flushed. My opponent appeared to be having a more difficult time. We each chewed, and I remarked how pleasant the chile was, conveying a delightful flavor as well as a moderate heat. The other fellow no doubt would have liked to offer an equally casual comment, but he was busy choking and gasping as tears streamed from the corners of his eyes and his nose ran. I finished the chile and inquired if he might care to join me for another. "No," he coughed, shaking his head vigorously from side to side. One was apparently enough.

The next day, I experienced a first-rate case of BSD, an acronym for a medical condition known as burning sphincter disorder. Experience shows that BSD is no fun.

I have, over the years, delved deeply into the physiological as well as the physical effects of chile consumption, and I can now offer some educated observations. First, you will find that some people like to engage in chile-eating contests. This is a mostly male, thoroughly macho inclination, and it is completely stupid and pointless. Even if you win, what have you actually won? The second observation has to do with the health and comfort of your posterior. If you like to eat chiles, avoid consuming the seeds. For while it is true that excessive consumption of hot chiles or their sauces will almost always produce some afterburn, this condition is primarily caused by eating the seeds, which contain high amounts of capsaicin. As the seeds break down in the gastrointestinal tract, they act like little chile grenades. This irritates the intestines, vigorously stimulates motility, and produces the often extreme burning sensation characteristic of BSD.

You cannot prevent silly men from engaging in chile-eating contests, but you can avoid, at least to some extent, the awful burning sensation that accompanies chile eating. Be alert—avoid the seeds.

Chiles and Health

As if chile reverie were not sufficient reason enough for us to carry chiles around the world and throw them into every cooking pot, hot peppers also promote and protect health in numerous ways. In traditional U.S. herbal folk medicine, chiles have been used to treat all kinds of disorders. From arthritis to asthma, colds to constipation, hemorrhoids to high blood pressure, lethargy to lumbago, and tonsillitis to toothache, chiles have played prominently in the formulas and practice of herbal medicine. Chiles have been made into decoctions, compresses, tinctures, ointments, and even vaginal boluses (ouch!).

In India's ancient healing system of Ayurveda, chiles are used as stimulants and appetizers, and to relieve dyspepsia, flatulence, lethargy, gout, rheumatism, sore throat, hoarseness, swelling, and tumors.

As researchers delve into chiles and their heat components, the capsaicinoids, their studies show that many of the traditional folk uses of chiles as medicines can be understood by modern scientific means.

Take chiles to heart. Chiles perform a number of functions that enhance heart health. They reduce platelet aggregation, the process by which disk-shaped structures in the blood accumulate and clog vessels. If left unchecked, this leads to atherosclerosis, or hardening of the arteries. Chiles are vasodilators—they open up blood vessels, thereby stimulating blood circulation and warming the body. Chiles help to reduce oxidation of LDL (bad) cholesterol, a primary risk factor in heart attack and stroke. They also reduce triglycerides, the stored fats in blood cells. All around, chiles are very good for cardiovascular health.

Burn calories! You're going to love this. Eating chiles actually helps you to burn calories and shed pounds. Isn't Nature grand? Research conducted at Oxford Polytechnic Institute shows that eating chiles increases thermogenesis, the body's caloric burn rate. If you eat chiles or chile sauce with a meal, your body will burn calories at an increased rate of about 25 percent. This translates into maybe 45 calories more burned per 700-calorie meal. That's pretty good. So splash the hot sauce onto your food. Crush chiles into your recipes. Eat it and weep. Burn the fat. Chiles are the hottest diet program going.

Possibly prevent ulcers. While some people imagine that chiles may cause ulcers due to their pungency, they appear to help prevent them in some cases. In one study, capsaicin prevented ulceration when excessively high doses of aspirin were consumed. However, most ulcers are caused by the bacteria *Helicobacter pylori*. While chiles do inhibit this bacteria in a test tube, they do not appear to do so in the body.

Fight cancer. Capsaicin in chiles fights cancer by preventing carcinogens from binding to DNA, where they trigger processes that cause lung and other cancers. This does not mean that chiles are a cancer treatment, but it does mean that eating chiles can help to reduce the risk of certain types of cancer, including tumors in the liver.

It killeth dogs, if it be given them to eat.
—Rembert Dodoens, 16th-century Flemish physician and botanist

Help halt headaches. Chiles provide relief for some types of headaches, especially painful cluster headaches. It may be that the consumption of chiles wears out the mechanism by which pain is transmitted. Some people take cayenne capsules for relief; several brands are available at health food stores. But you can also pour some hot sauce on food or eat a chile-laden soup. How do you spell relief? H-o-t.

Relieve pain. Though you may choose to reach for ibuprofen instead, chiles provide pretty good relief for pain. Chiles contain pain-alleviating salicylates, the compounds found abundantly in the natural aspirinlike willow bark (which contains salicin) and wintergreen (which contains methylsalicylate). Aspirin itself is a salicylate-based drug: acetyl-salicylic acid. Remember, when you eat chiles, you get a pleasant endorphin buzz going, which also helps to reduce pain. Instead of reaching for the Tylenol, try a habanero instead.

Open that stuffy nose. Chiles open up clogged and congested sinuses. If you have a cold or allergy accompanied by clogged sinuses, there's nothing quite like a steaming bowl of soup just loaded with fiery hot sauce to blast open your airways. Your nose will run like a river for a while, but then you'll be able to breathe.

Stop sluggish digestion and constipation. Chiles stimulate gastric secretion, which means that they get your digestive juices going. So if your digestion is slow or weak, a good dash of hot sauce in your food may prove useful. Additionally, chiles help to move sluggish bowels. While I have warned previously about burning sphincter disorder (BSD) due to eating chile seeds, I will amend my advice. If your bowels are clogged and you wish otherwise, sprinkle a good amount of chile flakes (crushed red pepper), seeds and all, on your food. The chile will act like a blasting cap; it may burn a bit, but it'll get the job done.

When Axi [chile] is taken moderately, it helps and comforts the stomacke for digestion: but if they take too much, it hath bad effects, for of its self it is very hote, fuming, and pierceth greatly, so as the use thereof is prejudicial to the health of young folkes, chiefely to the soule, for that it provokes to lust.
    —José de Acosta, 16th-century Jesuit theologian and missionary

Battle bacteria. Of the many health benefits offered by chiles, one of the most significant is their capacity to prevent food-borne bacterial disease. Pathogens in food can cause food poisoning, which debilitates the strong and can even kill. You may be asking yourself what all this protection against food-borne bacteria has to do with you. After all, if you live in the United States, the odds are good that you have access to a fresh food supply, and you probably enjoy the benefits of refrigeration as well. Nevertheless, countless harmful bacteria are found in common foods, and bacterial food contamination accounts for more than 3,000 deaths in the United States each year.

In a study published in the *Quarterly Review of Biology*, researchers examined recipes from 36 countries and noted a greater use of pungent spices in the cookery of hot nations. The hotter the place, the hotter and spicier the food. The researchers then tested a long list of spices against 30 different harmful bacteria that can occur in foods. The results were impressive indeed. Chiles killed 75-plus percent of the 30 germs in the study.

The agent in chiles that appears to kill bacteria is capsaicin. In another study, capsaicin was found to inhibit the rare but sometimes fatal *Vibrio vulnificus* bacteria, which is found in raw shellfish. Thus, eating chiles is not only a tasty and feel-good experience, but it defends your body against nasty microbes as well.

Boost beta-carotene levels. Chiles are exceptionally high in vitamin C and are also rich in the naturally occurring red and yellow pigments called carotenoids. Vitamin C is essential to life and helps to maintain both the integrity of tissue and the immune system. The carotenoids protect against cancer, stroke, and cataracts, boost the immune system, lower serum cholesterol, and protect against the oxidation of LDL cholesterol. Beta-carotene in chiles converts into vitamin A, which enhances vision. From a nutritional standpoint, chiles are packed.

Prickly Heat

As a rule, I do not write about my penis. Mine, or anyone else's, for that matter. Generally, it is a job better left to the X-rated vulgarians. But here, and strictly in the name of science, I must make a worthy exception. Follow along.

This incident took place back in the mid-1970s at a quaint and totally earthy crunchy natural foods store in Atlanta called The Egg and the Lotus. From the name alone you get the picture of what kind of place it was. We sold innumerable copies of *How to Get Well* by Paavo Airola, we stocked 200 different bulk herbs, and our completely vegetarian juice bar was a must-stop lunch spot for touring rock and roll bands and spiritual luminaries like Bhagawan Das. We were a hip, happening spot, suffused with peace, love, and pumpkin soup.

One day while I was working in the kitchen at the back of the store, an order of spices came in. Among the shipment were several strands of dried red hot chiles. A lover of same, I admired them and carefully hung them on a nail on a wall near the stove where they could be used one by one in stews and casseroles. A short while later, I ducked into the kitchen bathroom. (Yes, of course, I washed my hands—but *after*.)

I recall my brief days in high school football, and one moment on the field in particular after being kicked in the groin. It's a truly awful sensation, both sickening and disabling. And however embarrassing it may be to do so in front of an observant audience of friends' parents and female schoolmates, you wind up clutching yourself with your hands. You just have to. That's how the sensation felt as it came on in the kitchen. The pain blurred my thinking for a moment, until a searing and entirely local heat kicked in. *The chiles!*

I scrambled, hunched over, back into the bathroom, locked the door, rushed to the sink, filled it quickly from the cold tap, liberated my inflamed member, and sank it deftly into the water. And stood there for 20 minutes laughing like a fool. In retrospect, I should have known better than to handle chiles and then handle myself without washing first. But I learned a valuable and worthwhile lesson that I pass on here to you: Capsaicin has powerful topical properties.

In fact, capsaicin is so useful as a topical aid that it is a main active ingredient in several topical medicines. In the United Kingdom and in France, capsaicin cream is employed for the relief of neuralgia due to herpes infection. The capsaicin-based U.K. product Aradolene is employed for general pain. In the United States, the most popular physician-recommended topical remedy for arthritis pain, Zostrix, contains capsaicin as its sole active ingredient. Capsaicin appears in the German product Arthrex, which is recommended for topical relief of pain due to nerve, muscle, and joint disorders, and in Arthrodynat for joint disorders. Spanish preparations Balsamo Midalgan Compuesto, Killpan, Linimento Langal, Linimento Naion, and Linimento Sloan are all used for rheumatic and muscle pain. Capsaicin is an active ingredient in numerous Chinese and Indian topical preparations for sore muscles and joints as well. I have even seen capsaicin listed on the label of a sexual lubricant/excitant. Personally, I do not recommend it.

Kava
The Pacific Elixir

From the Pacific Isles comes kava, the peace plant. Kava is the name of both the plant and a beverage made from its pounded roots. Kava soothes. Kava rubs the sore and weary shoulders of humanity and eases the mind of its burdens. In this regard, kava is the perfect representative of the Pacific Islands, for it imparts to body and mind what the imagination conjures about all tropical islands. No other psychoactive plant so exquisitely complements the swaying palms, warm breezes, cheerful sun, and delightful blue waters that are such a part of island life. With ease and gentleness and grace, kava has captured those born to the islands as well as many who visit or settle there. Kava is an equal-opportunity agent of reverie, soothing and easing natives and nonnatives alike.

For 3,000 years, the indigenous people of the South Pacific have quaffed kava for its highly pleasurable feeling of tranquillity in body and mind. As a daily libation among native men and women, kava is most usually consumed at the end of the workday, and the ritual of kava preparation and drinking affords both a social time and an opportunity for individual reflection. Kava is nature's most perfect soothing plant. Consumed in moderation, kava is an elixir of peace, promoting a state of stress-free happiness and contentment. Many is the evening I have sat with friends for a couple of hours before dinner, drinking shells of kava and discussing the affairs of the day with a carefree heart.

In marked contrast to alcohol, kava does not inspire aggressive, boisterous, or violent behavior. It neither fuels arguments nor causes drinkers to say embarrassing or stupid things, and it doesn't produce any unpleasant day-after hangover. In moderation, kava does not incapacitate the drinker, hurt health, or fragment the mind. Kava is not physically addictive and does not diminish reason, mental clarity, or memory. Instead, kava's effects are essentially beneficial. Among the psyche delicacies, kava is the only one currently being employed as a significant medicine, even as a substitute for other well-established pharmaceutical drugs. Kava relaxes and refreshes at the same time. It promotes a good night's sleep and enhances vigor upon awakening.

Furthermore, kava is a social instead of solitary agent of reverie. Kava drinking reinforces social bonds, enhances sense of community, and encourages a spirit of conviviality among drinkers. Kava promotes togetherness, not isolation. In the islands, kava is used to settle disputes and resolve disturbances between people. Kava restores harmony, and even after the immediate effects of kava have worn off, the calm and sense of balanced reflection gained while under its influence remain. For a world that is cranked to the eyeballs with stress and tension, kava offers blessed relief.

The Legend of Kava

Pacific folklore has long associated the discovery of kava with sexual scenes. The most famous folktale concerning the origin of cultivated kava is the one that I'll now recount.

Long, long ago, on one of the islands in what is now Vanuatu, in the early days of the first ancestors, two sisters went out into the forest to gather wild yams for food. After collecting a large basketful, the women walked to the shore, where they could wash the dirt off the yams and scrape off their peels. The sisters squatted by a tide pool at the water's edge and began to clean the yams.

Totally unknown to them, a voyager from a nearby island had only days before secreted a special kava plant among the rocks at the water's edge, at the very spot where they were now working. While the two sisters cleaned their yams, the hidden kava plant sprouted a fresh green stalk that reached up and into the vagina of one of the women. Naturally, she was greatly surprised. She felt the tickling of the plant within her, which caused pleasurable sensations throughout her body. "Oh, my sister," she called out. "What is the agent of my excitement?" Her sister saw with surprise that a fresh shoot of kava was the stealthy agent of the other's sudden happiness. Clearly, this was no ordinary kava plant. They carefully removed the kava from where it had been hidden, wrapping it in a length of wet coconut fiber. The sisters brought the kava plant back home, where they planted it in their garden and tended it secretly for several years.

At that time, men drank kava made only from the roots of wild plants found in the forest and mountains. Sometimes the kava was pleasing, and it made the men feel relaxed and happy. But at other times the wild kava made them dull and caused their heads to ache. One day, when the special kava plant tended by the sisters was mature, the women dug up some of the root and presented it to the men at the kava drinking ground. "Try this," advised one of the sisters. "This is the true kava. If you drink from this kava, you will never drink wild kava again. This kava will give you the greatest pleasure."

The men were pleased at this idea and commenced to prepare the kava. For this task, they summoned a female virgin from the village. She was young and had dark eyes that would make a man feel carried away as if in a dream. She sat upon broad banana leaves and chewed the kava root very carefully, until the root in her mouth was mashed into a soft, moist pulp. She then spat the pulp gently onto palm fronds. After she made several piles of mashed kava in this manner, the girl placed the kava into a wide wooden bowl and added water. She worked the mashed kava in the water thoroughly with her hands until the liquid became the color of muddy water. Then she strained the kava twice through coconut fiber, poured the drink into coconut shells, and offered it to the men for their pleasure.

The men lifted their coconut shells and drank, one after another, until all had partaken of the kava. Soon they were smiling broadly with great happiness. They laughed and conversed with one another for a long time, forgetting all their cares. The men agreed that the kava cultivated by the sisters was indeed the true kava. And so it came to pass that since that time, kava has been prepared from plants grown in gardens and plots, and the men always chose it over wild kava.

The Peace Plant

The name *Piper methysticum* ("intoxicating pepper") was given to kava by Johann Georg Forster, a German botanist who sailed with Captain James Cook. A robust and attractive perennial shrub, densely foliated with smooth, heart-shaped leaves, kava is a member of the pepper family, whose 2,000 or more diverse species have been widely distributed throughout Africa, India, Southeast Asia, and Indonesia since antiquity.

Healthy kava plants are beautiful to behold, with variations in leaf color, from yellowish green to dark green. They typically have numerous stalks that arise from the root mass. Mature plants may have more than 50 stalks, which have nodes, or bulging joints, between stalk sections. The flowers of the kava plant are slender and green, and the root structure consists of a large mass or rootstock and a number of slender lateral roots. When kava is prepared for drinking, the lateral roots and the rootstock are both used. Of the two, the lateral roots are more potent, containing a greater concentration of kavalactones, the relaxing agents in the plant.

Throughout Oceania, kava has various names. In much of Polynesia—including Hawaii, Tahiti, and the Marquesas—the plant and the beverage are called *awa*. In Fiji, the name is *yaqona*. The plant is also known as *kawakawa*, a name derived from the Maori. In all cases, the name generally means "bitter." Kava is indeed bitter, and the beverage looks like muddy river water. Nevertheless, it is highly esteemed for its social, health, and magico-religious significance. In Fiji, Vanuatu, Tonga, and Samoa especially, kava and its preparation and consumption are central to society.

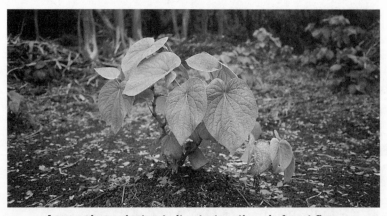

A young kava plant gets its start on the rain forest floor.

Piper methysticum is a cultivated variant of wild kava, *P. wichmannii*. Botanists believe that at one time all kava was *P. wichmannii*. As a result of cultivation, the plant in time became different from its wild progenitor, most notably in the root tissue. This is a common occurrence when a wild plant becomes cultivated. Cultivated kava is used for the preparation of kava the beverage, while wild kava is only rarely used, when cultivated kava is in short supply.

Researchers believe that kava is native to either New Guinea, the Solomon Islands, or northern Vanuatu, and that after its mind- and mood-altering effects became known, it was widely dispersed throughout the Pacific Islands by seafaring islanders. One thing is certain: Kava was consumed prior to written history, and its use was already well established throughout the South Pacific when Captain Cook made his first voyage to that area aboard the *Endeavour* between 1768 and 1771.

It is cool, refreshing, and stimulating without being intoxicating. . . . Used in moderation, it is probably the best drink for a tropical climate.

—Sir Peter Buck, anthropologist, physician, and politician

Kava is planted by various methods. In one, sections of kava stalks are laid in trenches of mud, where they sprout. The stalk sections are then planted in shallow trenches, where they grow to maturity. By another method, kava stalks are cut at a diagonal and simply planted pointed ends downward in the ground. Once kava is planted, its roots grow, sending up numerous new stalks above the ground. Thus, kava gardens and plantations grow perennially and are typically passed on through successive generations.

Kava plants mature in 3 to 5 years, though native people value older plants more highly for their greater root size and potency. By maturity, kava roots have typically become thick, knotted masses. The lush plant grows densely and is harvested when it is approximately 6 to 8 feet tall. Old kava plants can grow very tall, as high as 20 feet. In Hawaii, I have seen giant kava plants with stalks thick and strong enough to hang from.

Though kava is not cultivated on all South Pacific islands, it is found on many. Kava is grown on Papua New Guinea, Irian Jaya, Fiji, Wallis and Futuna, Western and American Samoa, Tonga, the Society and Marquesas Islands, Vanuatu, Tahiti, Micronesia, and Hawaii, where cultivated kava is making a resurgence after being considered a cultural relic for decades. Kava's widespread distribution gives testimony to the cultural value and social significance of this plant and its beverage.

Cultivation keeps growers, their friends, and communities well supplied with kava as part of a sprawling, increasingly lucrative agricultural enterprise ranging over thousands of miles of South Pacific territory. In the archipelago of Vanuatu, for example, large plots of kava are grown on several islands. From those growing areas, kava is distributed widely throughout the other islands and to the Vanuatu capital island of Efate, where it is consumed, traded, or shipped to other regions of the world. More than 150 kava bars operate in Vanuatu's tiny port capital of Port-Vila, whose general area supports a population of 20,000. An estimated 15,000 tons of kava is consumed in Vanuatu annually!

Kava cultivation requires relatively little labor or capital expenditure, and no chemical agricultural inputs. According to the Fiji Ministry of Primary Industries, kava is second in revenues only to sugarcane as a cash crop. Trade there is coordinated by the Fiji Cooperative Association in Suva on the capital island of Viti Levu. In the Republic of Vanuatu, kava trade is assisted by the Vanuatu Ministry of Agriculture and promoted by the Vanuatu Commodities Marketing Board. The South Pacific Commission is engaged in the promotion of kava throughout the Pacific, and even the University of Hawaii has taken a strong position in the promotion of kava, with agricultural specialists there helping growers to maximize yields.

Most cultivated kava is still used by native people, but the word is out about kava now, and an increasing amount of the root is exported for use abroad. French pharmaceutical companies have been purchasing kava from Vanuatu on a consistent basis for years. German botanical medicine companies have stepped up their importation of kava due to a sharp increase in use in Europe. U.S. botanical companies purchase kava from Fiji, Vanuatu, Samoa, and the state of Hawaii in ever larger quantities due to consumer demand for kava-based supplements. Japanese and Chinese companies now also buy kava. Thus, market prices of raw kava for export have risen over the past decade. In Vanuatu, exports soared from 50 tons annually in 1995 to 720 tons in 1998. In Samoa, the booming kava business has resulted in an increase in cultivation from 353 acres in 1989 to 2,600 acres in 2000.

Volcano Kava

Under tall coconut trees, four men sat side by side on a log, each with a cone-shaped piece of coral in one hand and a clump of freshly cleaned kava root in the other. Pressing the coral pieces hard into the kava, Michelle, Kami, Leno, and Jonas ground vigorously away at the tough, fibrous root, slowly and steadily mashing it into a fine pulp. Each one smiled and laughed as they toiled with muscular arms and the sun set, slipping below the far edge of the great Pacific Ocean, shooting its last rays of light out across the water in a brief green flash.

Sitting just outside of Chief Jean Paul's *nakamal*, a large bamboo hut built for kava drinking, the four men prepared the first few shells of the day's kava in the warm dusk. The kava for the rest of the evening would be mashed by pole pounding—and indeed the kava drinking would go on for several hours—but the men like to prepare the first few shells by the more time-consuming and labor-intensive method. The fine mashing releases more of the kavalactones, the relaxing active constituents in the fiber of the kava root. This method also wears down the calcium-rich coral, imparting a smooth, milky taste to an otherwise bitter drink. The fine, pulpy kava is mixed thoroughly with a small amount of water and then squeezed through coconut fiber twice, into a coconut shell. One shell of that kava is like three shells of kava at many kava bars. Very clean, and very strong.

The men were from the village of Baie Martellie, at the southern tip of the island of Pentecost, in the remote volcanic archipelago of the Republic of Vanuatu, deep in the South Pacific. Kava cognoscenti generally agree that in all of Oceania, the very strongest kava is made in Vanuatu. This is due to the fact that in Vanuatu, kava is prepared from fresh roots, whereas in other places such as Fiji and Tonga, kava is made from dried and powdered root. The men in Baie Martellie make some of the strongest kava of all, using little water and a lot of root. They say that the potency of their kava owes in

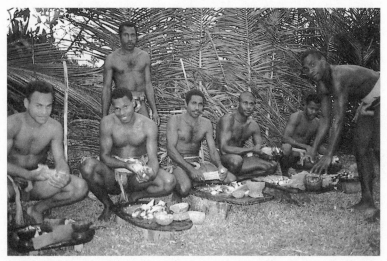

Proud kava growers of Baie Martellie make the finest kava in the world.

part to the varieties they grow and their methods of preparation. But they also insist that the mighty volcano across the bay makes their kava the strongest.

I first visited Baie Martellie in 1995, thanks to a fortuitous meeting with a Tahitian prince named Ariipaea Salmon, whom I know as Paea. In his company, we traveled down the coast of Pentecost Island to the village of Baie Martellie, situated on a spectacular crescent-shaped beach just a few miles across the water from the island of Ambrym, home of the gigantic, live Maroum volcano. Beautiful woven bamboo huts with thatched palm-leaf roofs lined the beach. The first time I laid eyes on Baie Martellie, I choked up with tears. Never in my life had I seen a place of such pristine beauty. Children played, dogs scampered about, and the place conveyed an overall joyful feeling.

Then the great tidal wave of 1999 hit. Three villagers were killed, and the giant wave smashed the village to pieces and washed the wreckage out to sea. Today, Baie Martellie sits perched high on a hill above that same beach, safely out of reach of any tsunami that might barrel into the bay. But it is still only a short distance across the water from the great and powerful Maroum.

The first night I ever drank kava in Baie Martellie, I walked out of the nakamal and onto the beach and stared with astonished awe at the spectacle across the bay. Fiery light from the immense cone of the volcano, roiling inside with molten lava, reflected an extravaganza of colors against overhead clouds. Out across the sky in all directions, gold, yellow, red, green, blue, and purple light spread like magician's smoke in great rolls. Majestic and powerful, the light and colors spoke of the enormous force of nature. Rising from sea level to nearly 4,200 feet, Maroum dominates Ambrym Island, and dominates as well the view to sea from idyllic Baie Martellie.

Most of the year, the tremendous heat funneling out the fiery cone of Maroum blows out on the ocean in a regular southeasterly wind. But periodically the wind shifts and Maroum's molten heat blasts full force into Baie Martellie. The villagers flee, retreating far back into the woods. They idle by the waterfall back in the forest and lie in cool streams until the wind turns back out to sea. The volcano's heat can descend on Baie Martellie for a week at a time. When this occurs, the entire bay heats up and the nearby hills cook. It is in these hills where the growers of Baie Martellie plant their kava, and so the kava bakes in the volcanic ground, becoming imbued with the elemental potency of mighty Maroum.

The growers of Baie Martellie will tell you that the heat of Maroum makes their kava more potent. Having drunk their kava many times, I can easily accept that claim. Drinking kava with native people anywhere in Vanuatu is a privilege and a treat, but drinking in Baie Martellie is something else. The spectacular location of the bay surely creates a virtually unrivaled splendor, and the kava itself possesses a preternatural power that weaves a hypnotic spell.

The head is affected pleasantly; you feel friendly, not beer sentimental; you cannot hate with kava in you. Kava quiets the mind; the world gains no new color or rose tint; it fits in its place and in one easily understandable whole.

—E. M. Lemert, sociologist

When Kami finished making the first shell of kava, he called to me. "Chris, you come drink." I walked over and picked up the coconut shell full of freshly made kava. I brought the shell to my lips, tilted my head back a bit, and drained it all at once, shaking the few remaining drops on the ground. All the men around me clapped. The day's kava drinking had officially begun.

Immediately after swallowing the kava, my tongue and throat became numb. The muscles throughout my body became softer, more elastic. My face became relaxed and pliable as tension drained from my facial muscles. I became aware of my breathing, which felt deeper, slightly more full and more pleasurable than usual. Over the course of the next few minutes, a sensuous wave of muscular relaxation washed throughout my entire body. My visual and auditory acuity also became heightened. I noticed subtle gradations of light and shadow. All the sounds around me became pronounced. The buzzing of insects was sharp and high, and I became acutely aware of the rich and varied tones in the voices of my friends. Meanwhile, my mind remained lucid and clear. The overall effect was one of delightful tranquillity and mental alertness. "You good?" Kami asked. I smiled and nodded in the affirmative. I was good.

Kava Cultivars

As is true with countless plants cultivated and consumed by humans, there are numerous cultivars, or varieties, of kava. In 1902, Western botanists identified 9 varieties of kava in Samoa. In 1935, 21 varieties found in the Marquesas were listed in botanical literature. By 1940, 14 Hawaiian varieties were known, and in 1984, more than 72 varieties were reportedly cultivated on the islands of Vanuatu.

The various cultivars of kava are distinguished by both their physical characteristics and by their effects upon body and mind. Kava differs in leaf shape and color, stalk shape and color, the distance between stalk nodes, and the presence of spots and other visible factors. What accounts for the differences in effects among various varieties of kava has to do with the concentration and ratio of the kavalactones. Some little-used varieties of kava dull the mind and stupefy. The most highly prized varieties quickly produce a relaxing effect that lasts for several hours, contributes to a deep, refreshing sleep, and produces no hangover.

Kava cultivars are also noted for their ornamental and spiritual worth. Sometimes cultivated to grow in specific shapes, kava is central to the rituals and various life passages of the people of Oceania. Thus, kava plants are exchanged and used at virtually all significant occasions and ceremonies.

Preparing Kava

Midafternoon at Ronnie's Nakamal in Port-Vila, Vanuatu, my friend Paea and I watched three men preparing kava for the evening's drinking. One operated a grinder that turned fresh, fibrous kava root into a pulpy mash. Two other men piled the pulped kava into rubber tubs, added water, and worked the mixture with their hands. Paea and I were there just to watch and take pictures. We would return early in the evening to sit and drink kava for a couple of hours. "How much kava do you figure is here?" I asked.

"I guess about 100 kilos," replied Paea. "It will all be gone tonight for sure." We both laughed, knowing how popular Ronnie's is. A nakamal like Ronnie's gains a reputation by serving fresh, clean kava, providing a friendly atmosphere, and being in an accessible location. Like a favorite restaurant, Ronnie's earns its good reputation every day.

On the various Pacific islands, kava is prepared by different methods. In Fiji, for example, dried root is used to make a mild, very light drink that imparts subtle effects. In Vanuatu, where I have spent most of my time investigating kava, the preparation is made from fresh root and the resulting beverage is appreciably stronger. The variety of species used is of primary significance. Some, such as the Borogu of Pentecost Island, are more highly prized than others. Upon chemical analysis, preferred varieties demonstrate higher concentrations of kavalactones, better ratios of certain kavalactones, one to another, or both.

Roots are usually mature and ready for preparing at 5 years of age. As time goes by and the root increases in size and weight, the concentration of kavalactones in the root increases. Kava roots can weigh anywhere from 20 pounds to as much as 100 pounds. Virtually every individual kava grower or village has a few very special plants that are 10 or 15 years old, saved for just the right occasion—perhaps a wedding, a circumcision, or some other important event. When a plant is harvested for use, it is uprooted, and great care is taken to pull up as much of the potent lateral roots as possible. The stalks of the kava plant are trimmed from the root, and then the root is scrubbed and washed clean, to ensure that the ensuing kava beverage contains no soil.

The potency of kava is directly related to the method of preparation. Mastication, or chewing, produces a stronger kava than pounding, grinding, or grating. Mastication may liberate more kavalactones from the pulp than other methods because saliva contains the enzyme ptyalin, which breaks down starchy components in the pulp. Historically, there is ample evidence that mastication of kava was at one time the method by which kava was prepared on virtually every island. Consider this firsthand account from the German explorer and botanist Johann Georg Forster, who accompanied Captain Cook on his second voyage to the South Pacific in the 1770s:

[Kava] is made in the most disgusting manner that can be imagined, from the juice contained in the roots of a species of pepper tree. This root is cut small, and the pieces chewed by several people, who spit the macerated mass into a bowl, where some water of coconuts is poured upon it. They then strain it through a quantity of the fibres of coconuts, squeezing the chips, till all their juices mix with the coconut milk; and the whole liquor is decanted into another bowl. They swallow this nauseous stuff as fast as possible; and some old topers value themselves on being able to empty a great number of bowls.

The notable exception to the practice of mastication was in Fiji, where pounding kava with a stone was the traditional method of preparation until it was replaced by mastication in the mid-1750s. Today, mastication is pretty much limited to special occasions on the southern islands of Vanuatu, notably the island of Tanna, and to parts of Papua New Guinea.

On some islands in Vanuatu, freshly cleaned kava root is placed in a standing vessel that resembles a butter churn. A length of wide pipe is fixed to a stump or other large piece of wood, and a heavy pounding pole is then used to smash kava inside the pipe into a soft, pulpy mass. In the nakamals, where large quantities of kava are consumed, meat grinders and even power mulchers may be used to transform fresh kava root into precious pulp.

Once kava root has been pulped, it is placed into either a large bowl or onto a broad, slightly concave board and is mixed with pure cold water. Kava is not cooked, distilled, fermented, or otherwise processed, but the amount of water used will determine the potency of the final kava drink. In nakamals in Port-Vila, quantities of 25 pounds or more of freshly pounded root are put into a large plastic tub and the tub filled almost to the top with water. Two tubs of this quantity will provide sufficient volume of fresh kava for dozens of people for several hours.

Once kava root is mixed with water, it is kneaded or stirred for a while until the water has a muddy, opaque, somewhat yellow appearance. After the kava has been thoroughly mixed, it is strained. In a modern nakamal, straining is often accomplished through the fine fibers of a sturdy nylon bag, but in traditional nakamals, the strainer used is usually a wide swath of palm fiber. In either case, the solids of the kava root are strained out and pressed, and what remains is a ready-to-drink kava beverage.

While some nakamals in urban areas now use glass bowls or other modern vessels for kava, traditional nakamals strain kava into coconut half-shells for drinking. In those areas where kava is consumed regularly, you will hear people say they had three shells or five shells the previous evening, or that they are going to have only two shells tonight because they must get home early. I always prefer drinking out of a coconut shell. The experience just seems more authentic, and I appreciate the feel of the shell in my hand.

In the modern nakamal, kava drinkers typically do not participate in kava preparation, nor do they necessarily even observe it. But in traditional village nakamals, kava is prepared by a few individuals while others drift in to share company and conversation and to discuss the events of the day. The men take turns preparing kava so that the burden is not left up to any one or two individuals. Energetic young men often assume the task of making the majority of kava as a contribution to the group, simply because they have the stamina to do so. Kava preparation is the beginning of kava time and determines the quality of the drink that will be shared, enjoyed, and appreciated. Because kava preparation is enjoyable to watch, I always prefer to drink in a traditional village setting. Many is the evening I have sat listening to the steady *toomp* of the pounding pole, and watched young men vigorously working and straining the kava. Usually, I am treated as an honored guest and can do nothing but sit and be served. But once in a while, the men let me pound kava, and this I enjoy immensely. Participating in kava preparation is part of the experience.

Kava's Battle with the Church

Each society has its own myths of kava origin. According to Tahitians, kava was introduced to the first people by the goddess Hinanui. For traditional Hawaiians, kava was a gift of the gods Kane and Kanaloa. And western Europeans . . . well, naturally they proclaimed kava to be the devil's drink.

Missionaries in the 1800s used the allegedly unhygienic nature of kava mastication, recounted by the botanist Johann Georg Forster (see page 136), as a rationale to press for a total ban on kava. Forster was a crew member aboard Captain Cook's ship moored off Raiatea when he witnessed two young men prepare and drink kava by mastication inside Cook's cabin. Even though the youths apparently exhibited profound respect for Cook and his mission, Forster was transfixed with revulsion at the native ritual. Forster's observations and illustrations of the plant set off a firestorm of interest in kava around the world, not all of which was favorable. As a result, native peoples were pressured to abandon mastication in the preparation process.

The journal entries of James Morrison didn't help the cause of kava outside the islands. Morrison visited Tahiti between 1788 and 1791 and offered this no-doubt exaggerated account of the effects of kava consumption on the native population:

> [Kava] almost immediately deprives them of the use of their limbs and speech, but does not touch the mental faculty and they appear to be in a thoughtful mood and frequently fall backwards before they have finished eating. Some of their attendants then attend to chafe their limbs all over until they fall asleep and the rest retire and no noise is suffered to be made near them. After a few hours they are as fresh as if nothing had happened and are ready for another dose.

Again, the idea of black-skinned natives chewing kava root into a pulp and making a psychoactive beverage from it was more than most white Westerners in the 1800s and early 1900s could handle. To many of the self-righteous Christian missionaries, kava drinking was seen as a devilish act. And like all acts of the devil, kava drinking badly needed eradication.

In the New Hebrides (now Vanuatu), Anglican and Catholic priests for the most part tolerated and accepted kava, even to the point of drinking it with the natives on occasion. But Protestant missionaries attacked kava with such savage ferocity that one is left wondering if they simply suffered from little else to do. The pleasure derived by kava drinkers so irked the Protestant missionaries that they became obsessed in their efforts to stamp out kava.

When the missionaries discovered that kava was sometimes used by natives to gain access to the spirit world, their antagonism toward the plant boiled to roiling outrage. Kava was an impediment to the establishment of God's law in a heathen land, they blustered. Kava ceremonies among natives often began with prayers to the natives' own gods for health, longevity, good crops, and success in various endeavors. The missionaries instead wanted prayers directed solely toward their own Christian god and wanted the peaceful sunset kava ceremonies replaced with repetitive, mind-numbing Bible study. Reflecting on the two choices, I have to say unabashedly that I would opt for kava every time.

The Presbyterians referred to kava as "grog," a pejorative term long associated with alcohol, and described kava drinkers as "drunkards." A pledge offered by the Presbyterian Church of the New Hebrides read thus: "I promise as a follower of Jesus Christ not to drink grog. When temptation comes to me I will seek the help of God's holy spirit." Dr. William Gunn, a medical missionary on Futuna, wrote, "[Kava] makes those who drink it drunk. Like alcohol, it does not equally affect all; but the drunkard from kava is intoxicated head to foot, body and mind. Though never hilarious or pugnacious, he is blear-eyed, staggeringly, helplessly, disgustingly drunk. Secondly, kava-drinking, as the natives themselves assert, is a heathen custom, and contrary to Christianity. Therefore, our members are all teetotalers." Actually, for the most part, the native people sought the gentle peace and help of the spirit of kava instead. But the Presbyterians were not to be deterred by the facts.

Marching onward as to war, the Christian soldiers implemented campaigns to eradicate the use of kava and were successful in some parts of the Pacific, including Tahiti and Kosrae. In Hawaii, the use of kava was banned except on the advice of a physician. In the New Hebrides, Presbyterian, Pentecostal, and Adventist missions attacked kava culture more successfully on some islands than others. In 1885, a meeting of all Presbyterian missionaries was held on Epi. Reverend Milne of Nguna made the following motion to ban all use of kava: "It be hereby enacted that no teacher connected with the mission be allowed to drink kava, eat things sacrificed to demons, or in any other way take part in heathen ceremonies." Not all attending missionaries supported the harsh motion, and this caused a rift in the assembly.

In 1886, strident Presbyterian exponents of kava prohibition went on the offensive again, and a convention of missionaries meeting on Tanna Island prohibited kava drinking for all teachers of the church. To the chagrin of the clergy, numerous individuals opted to continue drinking kava rather than to join God's heavenly legions and spread the joyous Gospel. This campaign against kava resulted in full-blown harassment of the Tannese people. Those who drank kava were threatened by the missionaries, and kava growers and drinkers were frequently arrested for nothing more than practicing their native custom. Those who were known or suspected kava drinkers were ostracized by mission members and were prohibited from attending church. Fortunately, they could seek soothing comfort in the calm peace of kava. The peace plant of paradise surely afforded more succor than the railings of the Church.

The subject attains a state of happy unconcern, well-being, and contentment, free of physical or psychological excitement. . . . Both natives and whites consider kava as a means of easing moral discomfort. The drinker remains master of his conscience and his reason.

—Louis Lewin, M.D., *Phantastica*

All this religious outrage undoubtedly had an effect on how kava was received and related to in the West. As proof, witness some of the distorted and deprecating accounts of kava drinking that were published during that dark period.

In the 1833 publication *Polynesian Researches*, William Ellis, a missionary in the Society and Sandwich Islands from 1817 to 1824, railed unrestrained against native kava users. "They were sometimes engaged for several days together, drinking the spirit as it issued from the still, sinking into a state of indescribable wretchedness and often practicing the most ferocious barbarities. . . . Under the unrestrained influence of their intoxicating draught, in their appearance and actions, they resembled demons more than human beings." Ellis exemplified the blind zeal with which many missionaries have attacked native customs deemed inconsistent with the principles and practices of the Church.

"Copious draughts cause a dizziness and a horribly distorted countenance," was the skewed view of kava consumption presented in *Torrey's Narrative; or, The Life and Adventures of William Torrey* in 1848. "They lose the use of their limbs and fall and roll about on the ground, until the stupefaction wears away."

In 1908, Sir Basil Thompson, in *The Fijians: A Study of the Decay of Custom*, delivered a strident indictment of kava consumption. "The body becomes emaciated. The skin becomes dry and covered with scales, especially the palms of the hands, the soles of the feet and the forearms and the shins. Appetite is lost. Sleep is disordered. Eyes become bloodshot. There are pains in the pit of the stomach. The drinker sinks into unwholesome lethargy."

A more balanced appraisal of kava drinking appeared in a Berlin Medical Society paper on kava published in 1886. The author was researcher Louis Lewin, M.D., one of the pioneering luminaries in the field of psychoactive drugs. According to Dr. Lewin, kava is "a real euphoriant which in the beginning made speech more fluent and lively and increased sensitivity to subtle sounds." Describing the peaceful effects of kava on drinkers, he added, "The subjects were never angry, aggressive or noisy."

Finally, in 1929, A. M. Hocart offered a sympathetic and accurate account of kava drinking: "It gives a pleasant, warm and cheerful, but lazy feeling, sociable, though not hilarious or loquacious; the reason is not obscured."

But then in 1948, Margaret Titcomb wrote a less flattering account of kava drinking, reportedly related by a Hawaiian named Kaulilinoe. "There is no admiration for the body and face of a [kava] drinker whose eyes are sticky and whose skin cracks like the bark of the kukui trees of Lilikoi in unsightliness. If you are drunk with [kava], you will find your muscles and cords limp, the head feels weighted and the whole body too."

A well-prepared kava potion drunk in small quantities produces only pleasant changes in behavior. It is therefore a slightly stimulating drink which helps relieve great fatigue. It relaxes the body after strenuous efforts, clarifies the mind and sharpens the mental faculties.

—Louis Lewin, M.D., *Phantastica*

Ironically, in 1900, at the very same time that kava was being bashed by Protestant missionaries in the Pacific, "kava kava extract" was being sold in the Sears, Roebuck & Co. catalog (#110) as "A Home Made Temperance Drink of the Purest Ingredients" and "the most healthful wine to be had at any price." The marketers at Sears went overboard, describing their kava as "exceedingly pleasant to taste." They remarked that their kava kava extract was "of great value as a drink for invalids, children, weak and delicate ladies, in fact, for everyone suffering from nervousness, low spirits or brain fatigue." Those who purchased a large package for $5.00 (about $100 today) received a set of six wine glasses and a decanter for free.

Meanwhile, back in paradise, the strident crusade against kava wore on. At the Council at Synod of the Presbyterian Church in 1947, a medical missionary named Dr. Armstrong prevailed upon the missionaries to pass a resolution stating "that since in the New Hebrides, kava is an undoubted intoxicant, and its preparation a dirty and unhygienic process, its drinking and use are therefore inconsistent with the Christian life, that it is the duty of missionaries concerned to appeal to Christians to refrain from kava."

At the General Assembly of the Presbyterian church of the New Hebrides in 1948, a further resolution was passed, stating, "The making of intoxicants inside the islands, particularly the notorious 'kava,' is to be discouraged as strongly as possible by all Christian workers. Office-bearers of the Church will abstain from all traffic in the kava root, and steps are to be taken to see whether the Condominium will make its use illegal."

The resolutions passed by the Presbyterians initiated a flurry of urgent correspondence with the British and French commissioners, who rejected a ban on kava as unnecessary and impossible to enforce. By 1950, prohibition efforts were abandoned; the Presbyterian missionaries were too whipped to fight any more. God's mighty soldiers had been repelled by a peaceful plant firmly entrenched in island culture, and kava had the last word.

Today in Vanuatu, Fiji, Samoa, Tonga, Tahiti, and other South Pacific islands, kava is experiencing an unprecedented resurgence. Churchgoers and traditional natives, many of them government officials and administrators, drink kava as an expression of traditional custom and as a way of relaxing, for all the beneficial reasons previously described. The tyrannical crusade of the Church is ended, and the kava-filled coconut shell remains both a punctuation to the end of the day and a means by which one may be conjoined with spirits and ancestors.

Kava's Tranquil Agents

Anybody who consumes good, potent kava can attest in minutes to the fact that kava produces a palpable, pleasurable, relaxing effect. This is the remarkable thing about kava. On many evenings in the islands, I have felt the relaxing "wave" of kava flow through my body even before the coconut shell has left my lips. Good kava is so immediate, it can surprise the new drinker. But what accounts for this? The active tranquility-promoting constituents of kava are a group of resinous compounds known as kavalactones. The kavalactones have been the objects of chemical research since the mid-1800s, and today much is known about their mode of activity. While as many as 15 kavalactones have been identified, only six appear in kava to any significant extent: methysticin, yangonin, dihydromethysticin, kavain, dihydrokavain, and demethoxy-yangonin.

The giant scientific step of isolating methysticin in 1860 opened the door to subsequent chemical progress with the resinous extract of kava. In 1874, scientists isolated a second kavalactone, yangonin, and in 1908, dihydromethysticin, the most active tranquilizer of all the kavalactones. Between 1914 and 1933, researchers identified kavain and dihydrokavain, and in 1959, scientists finally discovered demethoxy-yangonin. Today, the isolation and analysis of the kavalactones is made easier due to sophisticated methods and technology.

While the kavalactones were being discovered, their pharmacology, or drug activity, was of keen interest to researchers, and it continues to be so. Pioneering psychoactive plant researcher Dr. Louis Lewin found that injected kava resin produced temporary paralysis in frogs and sedated pigeons and sparrows to such an extent that they were temporarily unable to fly. When resin was injected subcutaneously into cats, the animals fell into a deep sleep. While these experiments may seem crude by today's standards, at the time they were ground-breaking and set the pace for further pharmacological investigation.

In 1959, researcher M. W. Klohs was able to demonstrate that there is a synergistic activity among the kavalactones that enhances their potency when taken together, rather than taken singly. This is not an uncommon finding, and it underscores an important point. The extraction and isolation of specific molecules from plants most often produces an inferior medicine when compared with the same molecules in their natural matrix of ancillary and related compounds. You can tinker with nature, but you can't do better. With kava, this means you'll get a far better effect from a concentrated whole extract of the plant than from its isolated compounds.

Thus, taken together, kava's tranquil agents produce local anesthetic activity with a potency similar to that of cocaine and procaine. Kavalactones numb the tongue and throat when kava is drunk in its traditional form or when taken orally as a liquid extract. First-rate sedatives, they produce a state of calm and promote sleep if taken in sufficient quantity. The kavalactones are excellent muscle relaxants and can ease the pain of an aching back, a sore neck, or any other cramped, sore, or injured muscle. They also have demonstrated significant antifungal activity against some human pathogens.

Kava as Medicine

For the most part, I prefer to drink kava in the islands with my friends. But there are those occasions, such as flying to a far-away part of the world, when swallowing a few gelatin capsules of kava extract helps to loosen my muscles, relax me overall, and make me more comfortable in a cramped or un-natural situation. And on many occasions, I have offered either fluid kava extract or kava soft gels to friends or associates with muscle cramps or spasms, headaches, menstrual cramps, or just plain daily stress. Almost without exception, they have found relief. This is the wonderful thing about kava: It straddles the line between agent of reverie and broadly useful therapeutic remedy.

Women going through menopause have told me that kava has evened them out, made them feel more in control. People I know who work in high-tension office environments confide that they keep bottles of kava in their desk drawers, to reduce tension when the day runs away with them. Parents and doctors have told me that, despite a lack of extensive scientific studies, they have used kava successfully to treat hyperactivity. There is a quiet kava revolution under way, a soothing medicinal sea change. Instead of reaching for a drink or a prescription drug, many people are turning to the peace plant of paradise for relief.

And why not? Kava plays a part in the native pharma-copoeia of Oceania, traditionally being used medicinally for a wide range of conditions. The primary folk medicinal use of kava is for the relief of urogenital inflammation and cystitis, for which it is still commonly employed today. But kava is also drunk to relieve headaches, to restore vigor in the face of general weakness, to promote urination, to soothe an unruly stomach, to cure whooping cough in children, and to ease the symptoms of asthma and tuberculosis. Applied topically, kava is useful for treating fungal infections and for soothing stings and skin inflammations. Kava has also been used to treat gonorrhea. Though no studies demonstrate efficacy for this purpose, prior to World War II, kava from Pohnpei was used by the Japanese for the preparation of a medicine used to treat gonorrhea.

Kava has also had a life in more conventional medicine. In the early 1900s, kava-based remedies made their way into the British pharmaceutical codex. In 1914, kava was listed in the *British Pharmacopoeia* under the name "kava rhizoma." Six years later, kava appeared in European dispensaries as a sedative and hypotensive. Kava also appeared in the U.S. Dispensatory as a treatment for chronic irritations of the urogenital tract. In 1950, the U.S. Dispensatory listed kava for the treatment of both gonorrhea and nervous disorders, under the drug names Gonosan and Neurocardin, respectively. Today, Kaviase, a French pharmaceutical product manufactured by drug giant Merrell Dow, is recognized by health officials of that country for the treatment of urinary tract infections.

I laugh when people make the claim that kava is "untested," or that its use for medicinal purposes is "too new" to rely on. This kind of uninformed commentary runs rampant through modern Western society and only shows how wholly brainwashed we are by pharmaceutical propaganda. Since when did centuries of human experience cease to matter? When you stand in a shower, do you need a double-blind study to know you're wet? When you get relief, don't you know it? Did you know that until World War II, a majority of medicines sold by U.S. pharmaceutical companies were herbal? Only patent law has changed that. There is simply more money to be made by inventing new drug molecules, however dangerous they may be. Kava, like so many other well-established botanicals in use for millennia, enjoys not only a long history of traditional folk use, but a long history of pharmaceutical use as well.

Nature's Answer to Stress

Kava's increasing popularity around the world is directly at-
tributable to the fact that no other plant or drug so readily,
easily, and safely dispels stress. Among herbs, kava is one of
the very few that you can actually feel the effects of. Nobody
feels ginkgo working in their brain. But you can feel kava, all
right. For this reason, dietary supplements containing effica-
cious, fully potent preparations of kava extract are available in
both health food stores and pharmacies. I personally am in
regular correspondence with many medical doctors around
the United States who recommend preparations of kava to
stressed and anxious patients before prescribing potentially
dangerous drugs. In the not-too-distant future, kava will be
one of the best-selling and most widely used herbs worldwide.
Almost everybody suffers from stress, and kava is the most effective stress-buster on earth.

Maybe we'd all be better off moving to Oceania, living
under swaying coconut trees, catching fish for dinner, and
knocking coconuts down from trees for a snack. Instead, many
of us live in a strung-out, anxiety-riddled world. As a result of
hectic schedules, financial pressures, inadequate sleep, family
difficulties, job demands, traffic jams, overcrowding, social
obligations, health disorders, life passages, traumatic events,
and other perils and pitfalls of living, people find themselves
increasingly stressed and anxious. The effects of stress and
anxiety can directly damage health, causing weakened immu-
nity, nervousness, indigestion, difficulty concentrating, sleeplessness, and fatigue.

The statistics are startling enough to make you reach for
a few shells of kava. According to the National Foundation for
Brain Research, between 17 and 23 percent of women in the
United States and between 11 and 17 percent of men suffer

from anxiety disorders. That translates to around 50 million adults in the United States battling anxiety! According to the National Institutes of Health Office of Medical Applications of Research, panic disorder may affect as many as 3 million Americans in the course of a lifetime. Additionally, an estimated 60 percent of American adults experience some degree of insomnia. Either they have trouble falling asleep, they wake up in the middle of the night and can't get back to sleep, they sleep fitfully and toss and turn, or they lie in an uncomfortable half-sleep and rise in the morning feeling dragged out.

To combat stress and anxiety, millions of people turn to drugs, both over-the-bar or -counter self-medications and prescription tranquilizers and sleep aids. Bad idea. Cheap and powerful, alcohol is the most widely used and abused antianxiety drug. Initially, alcohol can mitigate anxiety when consumed in moderate doses. But the longer alcohol is consumed, the more is needed to produce the desired tranquilizing effect. In greater than moderate doses, alcohol produces intoxication characterized by reduced motor control, impaired judgment, and aggressive behavior. Excessive use leads to addiction, liver damage, impaired brain function, and degenerative organ and nerve damage. Alcohol is the single most dangerous drug on earth, bar none. It is implicated in the deaths of tens of thousands of motorists every year, and it is universally known for its key role in domestic and criminal violence. Remember the Hippocratic oath: First, do no harm. Or, how about: You booze, you lose.

What about the use of tranquilizers, especially the benzodiazepine class of drugs that includes Valium, Halcion, Serax, and Xanax? According to their own promotional literature, these drugs may be addicting and may cause such complications as seizure disorders, vision problems, headaches, anorexia, neuromuscular difficulties, and psychosis. Habit forming, unreasonably expensive, and disputed from a safety standpoint, these drugs clutter the shelves of medicine chests and night tables of nervous Americans from coast to coast. Doesn't it make you wonder? The relief for a disease should never be worse than the problem itself.

Our minds are amazing, deep, and mysterious, rich with interesting psychic twists we're still exploring. One area of the brain, known as the limbic system, is a collection of organs that keys our feelings of fear, anger, sadness, and the myriad complex psychophysical responses that we call emotions. Homeostatic mechanisms in the limbic system regulate blood pressure, heart rate, body temperature, blood sugar, sexual impulses, eating, drinking, sleeping, and waking. Thus, thanks to shared neural pathways and other psychophysical factors, you can be anxious and depressed at the same time, experiencing fear and sleeplessness or loss of appetite and heart palpitations all at once. Drugs such as the benzodiazepines Deracyn and Zofran and others in development are prescribed for both conditions, then. According to the National Institute of Mental Health, during any 6-month period, 9 million Americans suffer from a depressive illness, costing the nation more than $30 billion per year. You have to wonder, when you read these gloomy figures, exactly who is healthy anymore.

In the limbic system, a small organ the size of a chickpea, the amygdala or corpus amygdaloideum—of which there are two; one left, one right—regulates feelings of fear and anxiety and processes memories en route to the cerebral cortex. This little organ is a primary site of activity for both the benzodiazepine class of drugs and for the natural, tranquil plant drug of the future, kava. Currently, the most popular drug prescribed for depression is Prozac, marketed as the cheery, feel-good drug to counteract every little psycho-emotional nuisance and dispensed by physicians like penny candy. Kava is the safer, cheaper, nonaddictive alternative.

Kava Studies

Millions of people over thousands of years have gotten profound effects from using kava. Among the five psyche delicacies presented in this book, kava is the only one with current, established, conventional use as a medicine. In order to move kava even further along the path as a beneficial alternative to synthetic drugs, it is valuable to know about some of the successful clinical studies that have demonstrated kava's beneficial effects.

- In a double-blind, placebo-controlled study of 84 patients suffering from anxiety, a daily dose of 400 milligrams of purified kavain (one of the six primary kavalactones) improved vigilance, memory, and reaction time.

- In a study of 38 patients suffering from anxiety, kavain and oxazepam, a benzodiazepine marketed under the trade name Serax, were compared over a period of 4 weeks. Both reduced symptoms of anxiety equally as measured by both the Self-Rating Anxiety Scale and the Anxiety Status Inventory. Oxazepam, unlike kavain, is addictive and produces side effects such as drowsiness, dizziness, headaches, and vertigo. This study makes it clear that kavalactones possess anti-anxiety activity comparable to the benzodiazepines but without the hazards.

- In a 4-week study of 58 patients suffering from anxiety, 29 were given 100 milligrams of a 70 percent kavalactone extract three times daily, whereas the control group was given a placebo. Those who took the kava extract reported a significant reduction in anxiety after the first week and said they felt markedly improved by the end of the study. As with other studies, no adverse effects were reported as a result of the kava use.

- In an 8-week study of 40 women with menopausal symptoms, half were given a daily dose of 100 milligrams of kava extract standardized to a 70 percent kavalactone value, and half were given a placebo. The group given the kava experienced a significant reduction in menopausal symptoms, anxiety, and depression, whereas the control group experienced no significant change.

- In a study of 12 volunteers, the effects of a standardized kava extract and oxazepam on mental function were compared. Using several parameters, oxazepam was shown to decrease both the quality and speed of responses to test questions, whereas the kava extract did not adversely affect mental function. In a word recognition test, oxazepam slowed reaction time and reduced the number of correct answers, whereas the kava extract slightly increased reaction time and recognition. This supports the oft-repeated claim of kava users that even when enough kava is consumed to induce a significantly relaxed, easy state, there is no impairment of mental function, including memory or clarity of thought.

- In a battery of tests given to 40 subjects, kava extract did not impair their performance while driving an automobile or operating heavy machinery. Unlike alcohol or the benzodiazepines, kava taken in appropriate doses (see "How Much, What Form?" on page 157) does not impair coordination, visual perception, or judgment.

- Two groups of 29 patients were followed for 4 weeks. One group was given 100 milligrams of kava extract, equal to 70 milligrams of kavalactones, three times daily. The other group was given a placebo. The study concluded that the kava was effective in mitigating anxiety and tension, without any adverse effects.

- Unlike the benzodiazepines, kava's effectiveness does not diminish over time. Whereas a person taking Valium, Xanax, or Serax may need to increase their daily dosage over time to achieve the same anti-anxiety effect, a dose of kava that works to control anxiety today will work equally well 2 years from now, one study shows.

- Kava is currently being investigated at Duke University and at the Columbia Presbyterian Medical Center in New York City. Continuing studies in those and other places will help to establish kava as a beneficial antianxiety aid without harmful side effects. The message is clear as a bell on a quiet day. Kava is not only good for reverie, it is highly beneficial medicine as well.

Kava Concerns

Kava is remarkably safe, but it is not a totally free ride. Kava potentiates alcohol, which means that alcohol and kava don't mix. Kava will make one drink feel like three. Also, if you are currently using antianxiety drugs or antidepressants, you should consult a physician who is expert in the use of kava before trying it on your own. We don't know all the interactions that kava has with other drugs. As a rule, pregnant and lactating women should avoid using kava simply to err on the safe side. There is no evidence of harm resulting from kava use during pregnancy and lactation, but better safe than sorry.

If used in great excess, kava can cause what is known as kava-induced dermopathy, a patchy scaling of the skin. I have seen this on some heavy daily kava drinkers, but I have never known this to occur among users of kava supplements. The condition appears to be harmless, and it goes away when kava use is suspended. I was once a guest on a national television newscast during which a very well known doctor warned that kava can cause yellowing of teeth, nails, and hair. This is a fantasy.

If you are going to use kava in large quantities for pleasure, I recommend that you do not operate a car or heavy machinery at the same time. In June of 2000, a man was arrested on Highway 101 in San Mateo County, California, after consuming 23 cups of kava. That's a hell of a lot of kava. He was acquitted because jurors were not familiar with kava. But in 1996, a Utah man was not so lucky. Weaving on the road after consuming 16 cups of kava, he was arrested and convicted of driving impaired. Be careful. If you consume very large amounts of kava, you may not possess the full faculties and reflexes needed for driving. Driving impaired for any reason at all is a bad idea.

I remember drinking too many shells of very potent kava one night in Vanuatu. I lay down in a little bamboo hut and listened to waves roar on the nearby shore as a tropical storm came in. Thunder and lightning crashed all around, and rain pounded down on the leaf roof. I felt as wide as the beach, as big as the night sky, and as out there as the stars. So yes, you can in fact consume too much kava.

How Much, What Form?

In 1997, the Kava Committee of the American Herbal Products Association (AHPA) commissioned a study on kava. The resulting report concluded the following: "Without medical supervision and advice, duration of kava use should be limited to a period of three months." The report does not suggest any rationale for this recommendation, which I find completely baseless. I personally know many dozens of individuals who have consumed great quantities of kava daily for decades without harm. The Kava Committee report further urged kava manufacturers to voluntarily recommend a maximum daily dosage of 300 milligrams of kavalactones on their product labels. Yet there is no research of any kind to support such a diminutive and restrictive dosage recommendation.

A single shell of kava as served in Vanuatu can contain anywhere from 150 to 500 milligrams of kavalactones, depending on the variety used, the method of preparation, the ratio of kava root to water, and the volume of kava per shell. Kava drinkers there consume anywhere from 500 to 2,500 milligrams of kavalactones per day for years at a time without any apparent ill effects. This casts the Kava Committee recommendation in a highly questionable light.

Successful human clinical studies show that a daily dose of between 70 and 210 milligrams of kavalactones can effectively mitigate anxiety in many cases. To promote sleep, a dose of between 150 and 200 milligrams of kavalactones taken 30 to 60 minutes prior to retiring is effective. But employing kava to mitigate anxiety or sleeplessness is quite different from using kava to produce a pleasurable feeling of tranquillity. In the latter case, the dosage consumed will typically be much higher. At natural products conventions, I personally have dispensed concentrated fluid kava extract in doses of 600 milligrams of kavalactones to several thousand people. Many individuals consumed several cups without suffering ill effects.

Unfortunately, many kava products on the market today are absolute rubbish. You get what you pay for with kava, and I want to caution you against going for cheapo, ineffective products. Only an *extract* of kava will relieve stress and produce a tranquil effect. Tablets and capsules of "kava herb," "whole kava root," or other ground-up preparations of the plant are a waste of time and money.

Look for kava extracts in tablets, capsules, or fluids that clearly state the concentration of kavalactones per dose. A single dose of kava extract in tablet or capsule form should deliver a minimum of 70 milligrams of kavalactones. Kava extracts in soft gelatin capsules will also contain oil or lecithin, both of which enhance the absorption and overall effects of the kava. A fluid extract should deliver 100 milligrams of kavalactones or more per milliliter. Avoid products that do not deliver at least these doses, as you will most likely get no effect.

There are other ways you can enjoy kava. Some companies are beginning to sell home kava kits containing dried ground kava root and a strainer. With these kits, you mix the kava with water, strain, and drink. In this manner, you can get at least some sense of the island kava experience. Another way to enjoy kava is at a kava bar. The first kava bars in the United

States have already opened in Hawaii. Over time, we will inevitably see a few in California. With any luck, we may even see kava bars in other parts of the country. Otherwise, it is truly worth traveling to the South Seas to experience kava in its native setting.

Kava Colada

On a warm evening on the big island of Hawaii, kava grower Zachary Gibson proudly demonstrated his latest drink, a kava colada. "See, I take a whole ice tray of frozen pineapple-juice cubes, put them all in a blender with a full can of coconut milk, add one ounce of fluid kava extract and just a little honey and vanilla, blend it all up, and it makes six really delicious drinks."

Zachary whizzed the concoction in a blender until the mixture was smooth and creamy. The fat in the coconut would help absorb the kavalactones in the kava extract. The pineapple, coconut milk, honey, and vanilla would all blunt the bitterness of the kava. Six of us hoisted the kava coladas and drank together. The drink was impressively delicious, and we all felt the effects of the kava immediately. Zachary was excited. "See? You make a drink like this with kava, and people will really like it."

We enjoyed the kava coladas so much that we made another blender full about 30 minutes later and drank those too. Half an hour later, we had a third round. Meanwhile, we did what islanders in Oceania have done for thousands of years. We sat together as the warm, golden sun set into the vast Pacific Ocean, and we shared thoughtful conversation and good company.

Peace Be with You

Every day we hear of people driven mad by tension, of ran-
corous disputes among the anxious and stressed. Every day we
are reminded of the wrung-out, fractious nature of the world.
And yet all social circumstances arise from the condition of
the mind. If people are thoughtful and peaceful, they beget a
thoughtful and peaceful society. If people are tense, anxious,
and angry, they produce a society that reflects their distracted,
fearful, and alienated mental state. This is the nature of
human life.

Kava is not a panacea for the world's problems, but it does
hold enormous value for those who wish to maintain serenity
and equanimity. We in the West have not yet begun to tap the
great and profound benefits of kava. For with this tranquil
elixir, the world settles into place, tensions ease away, and the
fundamental wholeness of all things is experienced. And this,
dear friends, is a good and precious thing.

Cannabis
Ganja Road

Cannabis is one of the most widely employed mind- and mood-altering substances on planet Earth. It is a sensuous magnet, a siren. An estimated *70 million* Americans have smoked marijuana: artists, laborers, lawmakers, poets, smugglers, diplomats, musicians, soldiers, sailors, actors, grandparents, hippies, rednecks, truckers, attorneys, physicians, journalists, holy men, freethinkers, buttoned-down businesspeople, and more—and virtually all of them, with the exception of President Bill Clinton, have inhaled.

Cannabis has spread all over the world from its origins in an isolated region of central Asia, despite harsh penalties in many places for its possession, sale, and use. Though not as widely traded as coffee or as broadly consumed as alcohol, cannabis occupies a distinguished place in world agriculture and commerce. Much of its trade history involves its use in making hemp fiber—perhaps the most durable and environmentally sound fiber product—for superior rope, paper, clothing, and sailcloth. But it is the psychoactivity of cannabis that concerns us here.

Cannabis delivers an expansive, spacious high. It heightens the senses. It makes music more rich, food more tasty, colors more vivid, touch more sensual. In some people, cannabis stimulates creativity; in many, it provokes laughter. The 1894 *Indian Hemp Drugs Commission Report* describes the effects of cannabis this way:

> Bhang . . . makes the tongue of the lisper plain, freshens the intellect, and gives alertness to the body and gaiety to the mind. Such are the useful and needful ends for which the Almighty made bhang. . . . Bhang is a cordial, a bile absorber, an appetiser, a pro-longer of life. Bhang quickens fancy, deepens thought and braces judgment. Bhang is the Joy-giver, the Sky-flier, the Heavenly guide, the poor man's Heaven, the soother of grief.

The healthful way to use cannabis is to secure high-quality leaf and partake of it moderately and judiciously. This formula for right userhood applies to the other psyche delicacies as well: Moderation, not habituation, leads to a maximally satisfying experience. If you resort to a joint first thing in the morning and rely on it throughout the day, then cannabis becomes a dulling habit that in time produces lethargy and forgetfulness. But used sparingly, occasionally, and in happy circumstances, cannabis increases pleasure and inspires a wholly embracing joie de vivre.

Of course, opinions about cannabis and its effects are highly polarized. Some people regard marijuana consumption as a fairly innocuous and pleasurable pastime that should be legalized without further ado, while others consider it a menace, an evil that destroys the mind and corrupts the fabric of society. One thing is certain: Cannabis is with us to stay. Drug eradication efforts have only invited cleverness on the parts of growers, dealers, and users. Cannabis use plays an increasingly important role in the ongoing human inclination to modify mind and mood, and a greater number of people than ever before in history are now more thoughtfully considering it as an agent of legitimate reverie.

Perspective

Let us lay a sober foundation here from which to consider cannabis. First of all, it must be stated that the war on drugs is hopelessly misguided as it applies to cannabis, which has been used by various cultures over several thousands of years and is appreciably safer than alcohol to both the user and society. The criminalization of cannabis makes felons out of many thousands of good and decent people. During the Clinton administration alone, nearly 3.5 million Americans were arrested for cannabis offenses. That's one American arrested every 52 seconds for possessing marijuana.

The unfortunate association with "harder" drugs is due largely to cannabis's illegal status and not because of its exaggerated role as a so-called gateway substance. In fact, users of cocaine and heroin typically begin their drug use by abusing alcohol more often than cannabis.

Decriminalization of marijuana would relieve an enormous burden from our law enforcement officers as well as decongest the courts, decrease the U.S. prison population of nonviolent offenders, get lots of guns off the street, and deflate a large sector of the illicit drug trade.

Penalties against possession of a drug should not be more damaging to an individual than the use of the drug itself.
—President Jimmy Carter

But let me be clear that cannabis is for adults, not children; that you can indeed use it to excess; and that smoking anything is not good for the lungs and the rest of the respiratory system. If you're going to smoke, then use top-quality, high-potency cannabis if at all possible so that you inhale less smoke for the desired effect. (The very best way to inhale cannabis is with a vaporizer, which produces an immediate effect without the tars and other compounds associated with burning plant material.)

Be responsible. Don't give cannabis to kids. *Ever.* Always keep cannabis, cannabis confections, and any other consumable product made with cannabis away from children. Use cannabis moderately and responsibly. Don't drive, operate heavy machinery, fly a plane, skydive, go hunting, or perform surgery or dentistry while under the influence. Don't operate a chainsaw after smoking. Do not try new gymnastics after smoking. Don't get your pets high thinking that it's funny. It isn't. Remember, using cannabis is illegal in the United States. Do not put yourself in risky circumstances where you might get caught. Keep your cannabis use private and controlled.

If you are going to consume cannabis by smoking, vaporizing, or eating it, remember the guidelines of set and setting. *Set* is your state of mind. If you are in a reasonably balanced mental condition, then that may be a good time to use cannabis. If you are feeling out of sorts, paranoid, or on edge, that is an excellent time to abstain. And don't rely on it to help you beat depression or cure your problems because it won't. *Setting* is your environment. Pick a nice place to relax, listen to music, or do something fun and safe. Above all, enjoy the experience.

Do not dare venture such an experience if you have some disagreeable business to conclude, if your mood is exceptionally dark, or if you have bills to pay.
—Charles Baudelaire, French poet and critic

Cannabis offers delightful reverie when it is used properly. It's great to be a psychonautic explorer, employing the expansive attributes of cannabis to generate a pleasantly altered state. But remember, you still live on planet Earth, so you need to follow all the rules of safety and responsibility. Cannabis does not appear to be addictive in the strictest sense, but some individuals find themselves sucking on joints morning, noon, and night. Moderate cannabis use is pleasurable, but dependency is not. Keep it light, and again, take to heart the words of Hippocrates: First, do no harm.

Just Say Know

Do government agencies suppress information showing that cannabis is relatively safe? You bet they do. In 1997, the World Health Organization circulated a draft of an upcoming report comparing cannabis to alcohol and tobacco. Using high-quality scientific methods and data analysis, the WHO researchers who produced the report found that cannabis fared more favorably than either legal drug with regard to long-term health effects. In five out of seven areas of comparison, cannabis was deemed safer. The report did state, though, that heavy cannabis use could promote psychosis in some susceptible people and that cannabis smoking "may be a contributory cause of cancers of the aerodigestive tract." The authors of the report stated that the comparison between cannabis, alcohol, and tobacco "was not to promote one drug over another, but rather to minimize the double standards that have operated in appraising the health effects of cannabis."

Much of the prevailing public apprehension about marijuana may stem from the drug's effect of inducing introspection and bodily passivity, which are antipathetic to a culture that values aggressiveness, achievement, and activity.
—*The New Columbia Encyclopedia*

The United States National Institute on Drug Abuse, the United Nations International Drug Control Programme, and a number of other antidrug agencies did not like WHO's message. Officials from those organizations reacted quickly to the preliminary report, urging WHO to suppress the document. Thus, a landmark study that physicians, health researchers, health agencies, and lawmakers eagerly anticipated was not released. It was a bad day for truth and democracy. When governmental agencies aim to suppress truth, they violate fundamental human rights. If life, liberty, and the pursuit of happiness are real and legitimate aims of a free society, then the flow of information must go uncensored. And if, as computer hackers say, the nature of information is to be known, then knowledge will reach people sooner or later in any case. Who is it that said the truth will set you free?

You Take It, and Siva Comes

The cacophonous traffic of Jaipur careened through the Indian heat in a swirl of brown dust as cars, trucks, buses, motorcycles, scooter taxis, ox carts, bicycles, cows, pedestrians, scampering children, and vendors of peanuts, coconuts, and rubber washbasins all vied for road space. Gaily painted trucks called public carriers were festooned like holy chariots with tinsel, colored lights, dashboard deities, sacred symbols, and paintings of the gods Siva, Brahma, Vishnu, Krishna, Ram, Lakshmi, the elephant god Ganesh, and the monkey god Hanuman. They groaned under impossible loads of every description, often populated by a clamorous crowd of Indians and their possessions atop perilously swaying cargo.

On that sunny November morning, I stepped cautiously to the edge of the road and hailed a yellow-and-black scooter, which jerked to a stop in front of me. "Where you want to go?" the driver inquired. "The Rambagh Palace? The gardens of the Maharaja? Perhaps to some shops with nice rugs or crafts or maybe some jewelry? I can take you to a good tourist restaurant with ice cream."

"I'd like to see some old temples," I replied after the sales pitch was finished. The driver fell silent and looked at me with his head tilted to one side. He tugged a corner of his mustache. "You don't want to go to the tourist places?" he inquired, somewhat incredulous.

"No, I want to go to some old temples, Siva temples." He

smiled broadly and extended an open palm. "You are a Brahmin!" he exclaimed, referring to the priestly caste that occupies the highest strata of Indian society. "My name is Sharma. I am a Brahmin too! I will show you the very best temples."

So there we were, Sharma the Brahmin and myself, thrown together by karma, the imponderable chain of cause and effect, speeding our way across the hot plains of Rajasthan province to the small town of Ajmer, where Sharma promised a very old temple built in honor of the god Siva. A complex god, Siva embraces all creation, all forms, and all potentials. This complexity is perhaps best described in the holy text *Anusasanaparva*.

> He assumes many forms of gods, of Brahma, Vishnu, Indra, Rudra, and of men, goblins, demons, barbarians, tame and wild beasts, birds, reptiles, fishes, with many varieties of human disguises. He is the soul of all the worlds, all-pervading, residing in the heart of all creatures, knowing all desires. He carries a discus, a trident, a club, a sword, and an axe. He has a girdle of serpents, ear-rings of serpents, a sacrificial cord of serpents, an outer garment of serpents' skins. He laughs, sings, dances charmingly, and plays various musical instruments. He leaps, gapes, weeps, makes others weep; speaks like a madman or a drunkard, as well as in sweet tones. He laughs terrifically. He is both visible and invisible, on the altar, on the sacrificial post, in the fire, a boy, an old man, a youth. He dallies with the daughters and wives of the Rishis, with erect hair, obscene appearance, naked, with excited look. He is one-faced, two-faced, three-faced, many faced.

Siva is the supreme god, the lord of the mystics and yogis. He is also the one who blessed humanity with ganja, a sacrament whose use opens the door to contemplation of the divine.

Sounding more like a lawn mower than a vehicle, Sharma's scooter taxi labored up a steep and dusty hill to an old plaster temple that commanded a wide view of the valley below. An ancient iron gate barred entrance from an inner sanctum, on the back wall of which a peeling wall painting of Siva spoke of the great antiquity of Hindu faith.

"This temple," Sharma explained, "is well over 600 years old. For all this time, people come here to worship Lord Siva." He pressed his palms together and extended them toward a worn statue. Near the front of the old temple, a huge terra-cotta plant pot stood more than 4 feet high. In the center of the pot, one very large cannabis plant with a stalk as thick as a broom handle rose proudly toward the sky. I gestured with surprise. This brought a smile to Sharma's face, and he wagged his head from side to side, eyes sublimely closed. "Yes, it is ganja, very holy. You take it, and Lord Siva comes."

The actual experience of the smoked herb has been clouded by a fog of dirty language perpetrated by a crowd of fakers who have not had the experience and yet insist on downgrading it.

—Allen Ginsberg, American poet

Many stories exist concerning the origin of cannabis. In one, the Lord Siva wandered out into the countryside after a family dispute (the Hindu gods have many dramas) and lay down in the cool shade of a lush cannabis plant. He ate some of the leaves of the plant and was so impressed by their refreshing effect, it became his favorite food. Siva subsequently became known as Lord of Bhang. Siva is also reputed to have brought ganja from the Himalayas to humanity to refresh the spirit, to allay fatigue, to erase cares and worry, and to provide human beings with a tool for direct experience of the divine, for general delight, for heightened sexual pleasure, and to bolster courage. According to other Hindu legends, the nectar of heaven, *amrita*, fell to earth from the sky and sprouted cannabis. Thus, cannabis, however it's called, occupies a sacred role in Hindu cosmology.

WAKE UP AMERICA! HERE'S A ROADSIDE WEED THAT'S FAST BECOMING A NATIONAL HIGH-WAY!

—Reefer Madness movie poster (1936)

Sharma drove me to numerous temples over the next few days. I spent the hot, lazy Jaipur nights in the quirky little Hotel Bissau, a small 12-room lodging that had served as a guest bungalow for the Maharaja of Jaipur during the era of the Raj. My room featured on the wall above the head of the bed a large, ferocious tiger's head with glaring, yellow eyes. When I lay down at night, I gazed up at the weird vision of a wild, man-eating beast lording over me with open jaws and sharp, flesh-tearing teeth.

At the end of each day, Sharma and I arranged our itinerary for the next. He arrived each morning, smiling and gracious, in a freshly pressed white *kurta*, a thigh-length shirt of crisp cotton, bearing the soul-satisfied expression of a man whose faith resides confidently in the unflagging grace of the Divine. I figured I could learn a lot from Sharma, and we gabbed incessantly as we cruised around. "I have spoken with my guru," he announced on the third morning. "He has invited you to his festival tomorrow."

The next day, Sharma's tiny taxi bore the two of us plus his guru, Maharaji, Maharaji's wife, and a large basket of goods. Also riding with us were Maharaji's slightly crazed attendant, Sri Ram, and a portly Brahmin with shaved head, heavy gold earring, and fine clothes. With four too many of us packed in, we sputtered out of Jaipur across the arid plains, eventually navigating a narrow, lonely dirt road. After an hour, we pulled up to a beautiful white temple compound in a remote and sparse place. At the front of the temple compound sat three men on a low wall. I sat with them and took in the clean but hot air and the steady sun, while Maharaji and his entourage went into the temple. One man produced a chillum, a straight, clay pipe tapered at the drawing end and wider at the lighting end. He pulled a clean handkerchief from his pocket and carefully unfolded it, revealing brown, caked cannabis. He tapped the chillum against his hand, knocked a small stone out from the tight end, and blew into it to clean out any debris. Then he dropped the stone back in and began to pack the pipe with the ganja. When he was done, one of the other men handed him a damp piece of cotton cloth that had been rinsed at a water pipe. The man with the chillum covered the tapered end with the cloth. The small stone would prevent embers from coming out the drawing end of the pipe, and the wet cloth would cool the smoke.

The third man produced matches and held one to the wide end of the chillum as the man who had prepared the pipe got it going. He puffed in and out with short breaths until the end glowed. Then he took a large drag and held it. The chillum passed to the other two men and then came to me. Cupping the pipe in my hands and creating a hollow chamber with my palms, I drew in slowly and steadily. The smoke was harsh, but not so much so that I couldn't hold it in. "Om Siva," one of the men said to me with a smile.

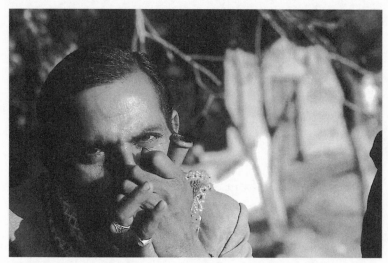

An Indian Siva worshiper smokes ganja in a chillum outside of Jaipur.

"Om Siva," I replied, smoke streaming out between my lips. It was the simplest and most direct initiation into the ancient use of cannabis as a sacrament. For Siva-worshiping Hindus, ganja is the bread and wine of communion.

We passed the pipe around until it was finished. I felt bright, elated, and spacious. Afterward, one of the men invited me to watch the preparation of the ganja. Dressed impeccably in a fresh, clean white kurta, he squatted on a long, flat stone. Placing a large pile of fresh cannabis leaves on the stone, he worked forward and back with another stone in his hands, mashing and grinding the fresh leaves. As he worked the stone, the leaves became mushy, and some juice seeped out the sides of the pile. He stopped to add a little cardamom and a small amount of black pepper and then continued to grind for several minutes until the ganja was a fine mash. Producing a clean white cloth, he scooped the mush into the cloth and squeezed out some juice. Then he folded the fabric several times into a neat package. He held it up. "This will dry in the sun, and then it will be ready to smoke."

People arrived seemingly out of nowhere for the next couple of hours, until the compound held a lively, bustling crowd. I wandered from group to group and person to person, chatting and taking pictures. For a while we chanted to a couple of men playing drums and cymbals. When it was time to eat, more than 100 of us sat in long lines and were served generous scoops of too many types of delicious—if unrecognizable—foods from buckets and platters onto our plates made of leaves. Sri Ram settled down beside me and probed into the pocket of his grimy kurta. He produced an oily wad of newspaper and unwrapped it to reveal a very large stuffed fried chile. Tearing the chile in half with his hands, he offered me the fat end, while looking at me in bug-eyed surprise, working the muscles of his forehead up and down. I laughed and bit into the chile, which was delicious. Sri Ram smiled, and I smiled, and we passed the day in Maharaji's company, surrounded by laughing children, turbaned men, and sari-clad women in gay fabrics until the orange Indian sun sank low on the dusty horizon.

Identification and Cultivation

Despite the best efforts of botanical experts to pinpoint the exact origin of cannabis, this information remains elusive. There is general agreement that *Cannabis sativa* is native to central Asia, north of the Himalayan Range. Botanist Gaspard Bauhin coined the Latin name in 1623, meaning canelike (cannabis) and sown or planted (sativa). Since then, many botanists have maintained that all cannabis plants are *Cannabis sativa* or sativa subspecies. But Russian botanists, as well as Drs. Richard Evans Schultes and LSD discoverer Albert Hofmann, assert that there are two other distinct species, *C. in-*

dica, or so-called Indian hemp, and *C. ruderalis*. *C. sativa* is a tall plant with branches starting higher up on the stalk; *C. indica* is typically shorter and more densely branched; and *C. ruderalis* is short and sparsely branched. Of these, *C. indica* is most consistently of high psychoactive potency.

Cannabis plants can grow as tall as 20 feet, with a furrowed central stalk from which numerous branches grow. The branches are covered with green leaves with long, toothed blades. There may be between 3 and 15 blades per leaf, though the cannabis leaf is typically represented as having either 5 or 7 blades. Virtually all parts of the cannabis plant above ground are covered with trichomes, or fine hairs. Among the various types of trichomes, those known as capitate glandular trichomes contain a resin rich in cannabinoids, the plant-based chemicals that produce the distinctive psychoactive effects of this plant. Cannabis plants are either male or female, and the difference between the two becomes most apparent at the onset of flowering. Males flower prior to females and pollinate the females as they flower. Then the males begin to lose vigor and wither, while the females prosper and thrive.

The flowers and leaves of cannabis plants are the parts that are smoked, eaten, or used to make hashish, which is the concentrated cannabis resin. Flowers, or buds, have a greater number of resin glands and are thus the most prized parts of the plant. Leaves of both male and female plants contain comparable levels of cannabinoids. But the flowers do not. In high-quality cannabis, male flowers can produce a high. But in lower grades, they may not do so at all. Female flowers, however, will be resinous and will produce a high. For this reason, growers apply their best agronomic efforts to increase female bud size and yield as well as potency. This is where the action resides. The techniques of cannabis cultivation are highly sophisticated at this point, and numerous highly potent hybrid varieties attest to the ingenuity of growers from British Columbia to California to Jamaica to Amsterdam to Nepal.

Fragrant smoke from the Arabian plant's brown juice creates a swirling dance of powerful fantasies.
—Moritz von Schwind, German painter

Cannabis is an annual herb. During the warm season, it grows from seeds obtained from female plants and then dies out. The plant grows in an astounding variety of soils and is decidedly not as fussy as coffee or cacao. Still, cannabis feeds heavily and takes a great deal of nutrients from the soil. The more fertile the soil, the better the quality of the marijuana. Cannabis maturation depends entirely on growing conditions and variety. Some hybrids can be grown to maturity under accelerated indoor cultivation in a scant 2 months, while others require as long as 10 months to mature; 4 or 5 months to harvest is typical.

To say that cannabis grows like a weed is no exaggeration. It does well in variable climate conditions (except frost), altitudes, and rainfall. It is generally hardy but can be damaged by wilt disease, leafspot disease, and branched broom rape, and young plants can be smothered by encroaching weeds. But although drug enforcement agencies around the world have attacked cannabis crops with alacrity, cultivation and yields continue to soar.

Nobody grows crops on a large scale like American farmers. In the United States corn belt, an increasing number of farmers are planting cannabis between rows of corn, perhaps due to low corn prices. The result is a massive tonnage of medium-quality weed. Corn-row cultivation represents a problem from a detection standpoint. Plots of cannabis are often located by aircraft using visual heat-sensing devices, as cannabis is a "hot" plant—it takes a lot of energy to grow and so possesses a strong heat plume. But corn is an even hotter plant. When cannabis is cultivated between corn rows, visual methods of heat detection are rendered useless, as the heat plumes of the cannabis just disappear.

Cannabis is a major outdoor crop in California, Hawaii, Mexico, Colombia, parts of the Andes, Jamaica and various Caribbean islands, parts of Europe, Turkey, Morocco, Lebanon, Afghanistan, Southeast Asia, India, and Nepal. Its indoor cultivation, however, is occurring almost everywhere that electricity and water can be had. In the Netherlands, indoor cultivation of cannabis is a multibillion-dollar enterprise. In British Columbia, the world's most potent superpot is cultivated almost entirely indoors. Cannabis is grown by millions of cultivators large and small. From New Hampshire to Madrid, people cultivate a few plants or a few hundred in indoor growing areas where heat, light, moisture, and temperature can be controlled to produce maximum yields and potency. Growing chambers, lights, timers and watering systems are available from garden stores and through various cannabis-related Web sites and publications.

Harvesting Good Buds

When cannabis has reached full maturity and maximum bud growth, it is ready for harvesting. After the main stalk is cut in a way that is similar to chopping down a tree, the plant is dried, usually by hanging it upside down. When the plants are dry, the lateral branches are cut from the main stalk and the buds and leaf material are picked from branches and stems.

Trimming is a key aspect of post-harvest processing. People do not want to pay for stems and stalks. Cannabis is expensive—and sold by weight—and there is no point in paying for parts of the plant that cannot be used. The trimming process results in a higher concentration of consumable material and less waste.

O Great Hashish

At the Jaynti Mata Temple in Someshwar, in the Kumaon district of the Indian Himalayas, the priest Gopal Giri Mahatma invited me to join in worship of Siva. "Smoking?" he asked, leaning toward me on the tiger skin where he sat. I said I would be happy to join him. He produced a folded piece of paper in which he kept chopped charas, the regional hashish. Gopal Giri Mahatma handed the charas to me along with a cigarette, which I emptied of tobacco and filled carefully with the sacrament. "Om Siva," the priest offered as I lit the ganja. I replied in kind. We sat together and smoked and then passed a pleasant hour or so in the shade as birds fluttered about and a small *dhuni*, or holy fire, burned next to us. This scene is repeated in Himalayan temples every day. Priests and pilgrims sit together, take holy communion in the form of charas, and bask in the grace of Siva. The tradition goes back many centuries.

Hashish is the most potent and concentrated form of cannabis, the pressed resin glands of mature female cannabis flowers. When cannabis is mature and the buds are sticky with pregnant resin glands, then hashish can be made by various methods. In the Himalayan foothills of India and Nepal, collectors run their hands up and down against the resinous flowers of mature plants until their palms are covered with resin. They then rub their hands vigorously together to clump the resin into little balls, which are rubbed together into larger balls or into "fingers" of charas. This charas is fragrant and sweet, with a floral aroma, conveying a pleasant, lively high. As romantic as the hand-rubbing method of hashish production may seem, it is very inefficient and really only suitable for those instances in which there is a large amount of ganja available. This is certainly the case in the Himalayan foothills, where the yards of most homes feature a plot of cannabis for charas, hemp fiber, and nutritious seeds for cooking. The people in that region enjoy a superabundance of high-quality cannabis.

In Central India, the hemp resin called churrus is collected during the hot season in the following manner. Men clad in leathern dresses run through the hemp fields, brushing through the plants with all possible violence; the soft resin adheres to the leather, and is subsequently scraped off and kneaded into balls.

—Mordecai Cubitt Cooke, 19th-century British mycologist and phycologist

For the most part, though, hashish is made by sieving. In this method, ripe cannabis plants are harvested, and when they are reasonably dry, they are then shaken or lightly beaten against a fine sieve through which the tiny resin glands fall. This results in a pile of fine, dustlike resin that is highly malleable and easily molded at room temperature. The resin may be rolled into balls by hand, hammered into concentrated blocks, or mechanically pressed into squares.

Some old methods of hashish manufacture involve rubbing the plants against coarse carpet before sieving, or sieving through fine cloth. The important part of the process is that as much resin as possible is collected, and after that, any pieces of leaf or other debris are removed by the sieve. Fine-quality hashish is free of debris, contains no mold, is uniform in color and texture, and is malleable in the hand at room temperature.

Different regions produce different types of hashish. The legendary Nepalese Temple Ball and Manali cream varieties are both black and smooth. Hashish from the Bekaa Valley in Lebanon is often red. Most Afghani hash is greenish brown. Some Middle Eastern hashish is blond or pink. Some hashish is even stamped with a seal of origin. I remember hashish in the early 1970s stamped with the gold seal of the Afghani Resistance. Whatever the type or the origin, the goal of any real quality maker of hashish is to produce a uniform product made solely from resin glands, to ensure purity and potency.

Not being used to hashish . . . he burst into extraordinary hilarity and filled the hall with shouts of laughter. A moment later he collapsed backward onto the marble floor and fell prey to hallucinations.
—*The Arabian Nights*, "The Tale of the Hashish Eater"

All things considered, hashish is the cognac of ganja products. Throughout much of India, Nepal, Kashmir, Turkey, and the Middle East, hashish is the preferred form of cannabis. This preference is owed to its rarefied nature and exquisite effects.

Hashish is either smoked in a pipe or eaten. As a smoke, it is typically pleasant and lofty. Eaten, it can be wildly powerful. (See "Maximizing Cannabis Potency" on page 199.) Beware, though. Hashish is most often made in conditions where hygiene and sanitation are poor. Pathogenic bacteria can and do reside in hash. You can become very sick from these bacteria, so you should approach the eating of hashish with caution. *Be sure to cook it.*

A shock, as of some unimagined vital force, shoots without warning through my entire frame, leaping from my fingers' ends, piercing my brain, startling me till I nearly spring from my chair.

—Fitz Hugh Ludlow, *The Hasheesh Eater*

In some places, you can find hashish oil. This is a product made by extracting the oily cannabinoids from hashish with hydrocarbon solvents. Depending on whether filtration is part of the procedure, the resulting oily goo can be black or even amber colored, as in the so-called honey oil of Nepal. Hash oil has never really caught on widely, most probably because it is sticky, messy to use, and not really necessary. It is, however, extremely potent. But well-made hashish is consistently more fragrant and enjoyable and far easier to use.

Cannabis Travels

Like the other psyche delicacies, cannabis has traveled far and wide. One historical account states that in ancient times an Indian pilgrim introduced cannabis use to Khorasan (northeastern Iran). From there, cannabis spread to Chaldea (southernmost valley of the Tigris and Euphrates rivers), into Syria, Egypt, and Turkey. It's most likely been a companion of humans since the advent of agriculture, around 10,000 years ago. It has been cultivated for its fiber, its oil, its nutritious seeds, and its psychoactive buds.

Hemp fibers thousands of years old have been found in China. The emperor and revered herbalist Shen Nung wrote about cannabis in the 28th century B.C., recommending its use for rheumatic pain, constipation, and female "disorders." He commented that cannabis "makes one communicate with spirits and lightens one's body." Cannabis was also used in Chinese magical ceremonies for divination. Later, around A.D. 200, the herbalist and surgeon Hua Tuo employed cannabis in wine as an anesthetic.

In India, cannabis fit well into the traditional folk medicine. The plant was referred to in the ancient *Artha Veda*, which may have been written as early as the treatise by Shen Nung. The plant was recommended for a variety of health needs, from relieving dysentery and improving digestion to easing headache and improving judgment. The *Rajanirghanta*, penned around the year 300, recommended cannabis to alleviate flatulence, stimulate appetite, and boost memory. Later, the *Tajni Guntu* described cannabis as a strengthener, a promoter of success, a mover of laughter, and a sexual excitant. In the Hindu tantras, cannabis was described as an empowering intoxicant. The plant was made into "pills of gaiety." Its psychoactive properties gave cannabis high status as a divine elixir, a life-promoting, soul-vitalizing agent. In the Indian Himalayan and the Tibetan plateaus, cannabis achieved high religious esteem.

I advise any bashful young man to take hashish when he wants to offer his heart to any fair lady, for it will give him the courage of a hero, the eloquence of a poet, the ardor of an Italian.

—Louisa May Alcott, "Perilous Play"

Archaeological evidence shows that the Assyrians used cannabis for incense during the first millennium B.C. Hair analysis of Egyptian mummies dating back to 1070 B.C. reveals high levels of cannabis residue, which puts the spread of cannabis into Egypt prior to that time. Hashish became especially popular, spreading throughout Asia Minor during the first millennium A.D., and from there into Africa. Early Arabian manuscripts describe the Garden of Cafour near Cairo as a major location for the use of hashish by fakirs. Tribespeople in Africa, notably the Bushmen, Kaffirs, and Hottentots (who called cannabis *dacha*), embraced the euphoria-producing effects of cannabis. The plant was used enthusiastically throughout Africa.

Cannabis may even have been mentioned as *pannag* in the Bible, in Ezekiel 27:17. Pannag is linguistically similar to the Sanskrit *bhang*. Are the visions of Ezekiel the psychedelic results of cannabis consumption? In Jerusalem, remains of burned cannabis show its use there around A.D. 400.

Sometime around 450 B.C., the Greek historian Herod-
otus recounted the use of cannabis by Scythian horsemen in
central Asia:

> They make a booth by fixing in the ground three sticks in-
> clined toward one another, and stretching around them
> woolen felts, which they arrange so as to fit as close as pos-
> sible: Inside the booth a dish is placed upon the ground,
> into which they put a number of red-hot stones and then
> add some hemp seed. . . . The Scythians, as I said, take
> some of this hemp-seed, and, creeping under the felt cov-
> erings, throw it upon the red-hot stones; immediately it
> smokes and gives out such a vapor as no Grecian vapor bath
> can exceed: the Scyths, delighted, shout for joy.

This account has been confirmed in archaeological digs,
with the discovery of an apparatus as described. However,
residues show that cannabis leaves and buds were the materials that produced Scythian euphoria, not the seeds. The
Scythians took cannabis, their joy-giver, across Asia westward
to Europe. An urn found in Berlin and dated around 500 B.C.
contained cannabis leaves and seeds. Within a short period,
cannabis had made its way to England, Scotland, and Ireland.

In A.D. 200, Greco-Roman physician Galen wrote that
hemp was sometimes given to guests for their enjoyment, and
Pliny the Elder mentioned cannabis in his *Naturalis Historia*
in A.D. 77. But cannabis became an item of value in early Europe primarily for its fiber. Merry olde England took up
cannabis with vigor during the Anglo-Saxon period from A.D.
400 to 1100. The plant was produced on a large scale for its
fiber. The superiority of hemp fiber for maritime purposes
ensured not only that cannabis would sail the seas among the
seafaring explorers and traders of Europe, but also that its cultivation would be spread far and wide.

In the 13th century, Marco Polo recounted the tale of the hashishan, or assassins, who were followers of a mysterious "Old Man of the Mountain." According to history, the warlord Hasan ibn al-Sabah resided in the mountain fortress of Alamut, south of the Caspian Sea. Hasan ibn al-Sabah reputedly intoxicated young recruits with hashish and indulged them with women and all manner of pleasures. Informing the soldiers that such rewards would be theirs as a result of unwavering service to him, he garnered extreme loyalty among his troops. The young hashishan were bold, fierce, fearless, and willing to sacrifice themselves for their leader's cause, assured of a hash-intoxicated idyllic afterlife. The assassins spread throughout Persia and Syria, becoming a much feared sect.

By God, bravo, hashish! It stirs deep meanings. Don't pay attention to those who blame it. Refrain from the daughter of the vines. And do not be stingy with it. Eat it dry always and live! By God, bravo, hashish!

It is above pure wine. When noble men use it, eat and agree, young man. Eating it revives the dead. By God, bravo, hashish!

It gives the stupid, inexperienced, dull person the cleverness of a straightforward sage. I don't think I can escape from it.

By God, bravo, hashish!

—from a 13th-century Arabian tale

In a parallel time, cannabis was making its way across the Atlantic to the West. Historical record shows that Spanish sailors introduced cannabis to Chile in 1545 and to Peru in 1554. Analysis of Peruvian mummies dated between A.D. 200 and 1500, however, shows traces of cannabis, which suggests earlier contact between the Americas and Asia or Egypt. African slaves who arrived in South America in the 17th and 18th centuries contributed to the spread of cannabis in that region, for in their homeland, cannabis was already widely used.

British sailors dutifully delivered cannabis to Canada in 1606 and to Virginia in 1611. In 1632, the Pilgrims brought cannabis to New England, but the low-resin cannabis was used for hemp fiber, not euphoria. While hemp was made into rope in the north, things were a bit different south of the border. Cannabis was used for psychoactive purposes by the Tepecano Indians of northwest Mexico, and migrant Mexican laborers introduced marijuana smoking to the southwestern United States. These laborers, as well as African slaves, established cannabis use in the American South. The famous English explorer Sir Richard Francis Burton wrote in 1885, "I found the drug well known to the Negroes of the Southern United States and of Brazil, although few of their owners had ever heard of it." From its agricultural roots in the Southwest and the Deep South, cannabis smoking spread to the jazz world in New Orleans and from there to numerous cities in the United States.

In the 1840s, French doctor Jacques-Joseph Moreau published several papers on the use of cannabis for mental illness. His 1845 publication *Hashish and Mental Illness; Psychological Studies* sparked great interest in the use of cannabis and its concentrated resin. In 1846, Moreau and Théophile Gautier established Le Club des Haschischins (The Hashish Users' Club). With its exotic drug and Arabian theme, the club became a hot spot for writers, including Alexandre Dumas,

Honoré de Balzac, Charles Baudelaire, and numerous others. This concrescence of hashish and the literati sparked a profusion of literary accounts of cannabis use and greatly popularized the plant and its use among the cognoscenti. Hoisted high on the shoulders of some of the greatest literary figures of that time, cannabis became an exotic cause célèbre.

Taken moderately, hashish cheers a person's mind, and at most, perhaps, induces him to untimely laughing. If larger doses are taken, producing the so-called fantasia, we are seized by a delightful sensation that accompanies all the activities of our mind. It is as if the sun were shining on every thought passing through our brain, and every movement of our body is a source of delight.

—Dr. Jacques-Joseph Moreau

Since its first use by humans thousands of years ago, cannabis has proven to be an unstoppable force. Eradication efforts have failed miserably, as they run counter to the natural human tendency to seek satisfying pleasure through friendly plants. In 1378, the Arabian Emir Soudoun Sheikouni placed a ban on the use of cannabis and imposed penalties and imprisonment for its use. Despite this ban, cannabis use flourished unabated. This is the first known ban on cannabis, which would be repeatedly insulted in this manner throughout history.

In 1894, the British government, concerned over widespread cannabis use in its colony of India, commissioned the now famous seven-volume *Indian Hemp Drugs Commission Report*. This extensive survey detailed the history and use of cannabis throughout the Indian subcontinent and its people. The report concluded that cannabis use was of little concern to health, and that "moderate use of hemp drugs produces no injurious effects on the mind."

Intense anticannabis crusading in the United States in the 1930s made the plant illegal in October 1937. Despite penalties, cannabis use continued to expand. Marijuana smoking was embraced by members of the 1950s Beat movement, including Jack Kerouac, Allen Ginsberg, William S. Burroughs, Neal Cassady, and other influential literary figures.

With my inexhaustible supply of Elitch [cannabis], I daily dive into these dim regions and crawl to the surface with the stub of a pencil, sweating, to record what I have observed.
—Jack Kerouac, writer, wanderer, psyche argonaut

Marijuana became the burning emblem of the hippie era of the 1960s, a revolutionary handoff from the Beats. Pot made people open and receptive. It encouraged frivolity and the free expression of new ideas. Pot was more than a substance. It stood for peace and love and freedom. It was a brick thrown through the plateglass window of stifling social conservatism. It was a statement about the kind of expansive experiences people could share. Pot smoking spread across the nation, as millions turned on with cannabis and psychedelic rock music. That explosion reverberated throughout the world.

Since the 1960s, cannabis has become increasingly popular. The growth of the Rastafarian movement in Jamaica not only further popularized cannabis but also produced reggae, a vastly popular, ganja-inspired musical genre. Today, cannabis is well-loved and widely employed by hundreds of millions of people worldwide.

THC, the Big Kahuna

Cannabis produces its satisfying and euphoric effects thanks to THC, or tetrahydrocannabinol, which is found in the cannabis resin. This compound is a member of a group of compounds known as the cannabinoids. Of these, more than 70 are currently known. But it is the THC content alone that determines the potency of the cannabis.

It is no surprise to discover that the brain is uniquely fitted to accommodate the active constituents of marijuana. In 1990, researchers reported in the journal *Nature* the discovery of receptors in the brain that specifically accommodate the cannabinoids in pot. THC binds to unique receptor sites, as though the brain were specifically designed to utilize this plant, producing euphoria and relaxation. Did nature toss cannabinoid receptors into the brain by random chance? Are these physical structures accidental neurological junk? Or are cannabinoid receptors part of an intelligent design for deriving maximum benefit from cannabis?

The acute toxicity of THC is extremely low, and there has never been a reported case of a death due to cannabis consumption in any form. THC is lyophilic and thus mixes well with various oils. For this reason, THC is readily dispersible in butter and other fats used in the making of baked goods and confections.

THC is rapidly absorbed, and its various metabolites are eventually excreted. But THC remains in tissues for a while and can be detected in urine a week or more after consumption. THC has also been isolated and purified into a prescription anti-emetic drug, Marinol, which is available in 2.5-, 5-, and 10-milligram oral doses. But Marinol does not produce the pleasures of cannabis consumption.

I began to gather the leaves of this plant and to eat them, and they have produced in me the gaiety that you witness. Come with me, then, that I may teach you to know it.

—Andrew Kimmons, *Tales of Hashish*

Cannabis today is a heck of a lot more potent than it used to be. As cultivation has become increasingly sophisticated, the concentration of THC has increased significantly. In the late 1960s, pot contained on average between 2 and 4 percent THC. Today, specialty hybrid varieties hit an impressive 15 percent or higher, and the British Columbian superweed has set a new standard at a whopping 30 percent THC by weight.

Cannabis as Medicine

In 1978, while working as a furniture mover, I broke my seventh cervical vertebra. The injury was quite serious and caused me chronic pain for an extended period of time. Often the pain was so excruciating that I could not move. I tried Tylenol, which did nothing. Acupuncture and chiropractic offered only temporary relief. I found that if I sat still in the lotus position for an hour or more, I could reduce the pain. Nothing else seemed to help. But this method was a bit impractical. Then a friend suggested that I try smoking marijuana. "It will get rid of the pain," he asserted. I was totally skeptical.

I had stopped using marijuana 7 years prior to that and had no particular interest in taking it up again. I was surprised, too, by my friend's assertion that pot would ease my pain. But I was desperate, so I tried smoking some. After just a couple of tokes, the pain began to subside. I found blessed relief. As a result of the judicious and controlled use of cannabis, I was able to move about with a minimum of discomfort, almost entirely free of pain. I could work a full day and was able to meet all my responsibilities with my usual high level of energy and care. The treatment was a resounding success. As a result of that experience, I will say that the controversy over whether marijuana is an effective pain-relieving agent is propagated only by those who have never tried it. Pompous pedants postulate and ponder and foot-drag over cannabis. But the results are very straightforward. Cannabis relieves pain, in many cases quickly and easily. For me, cannabis turned out to be a godsend. I became functional instead of bedridden.

Cannabis has been employed as a valuable medicine since antiquity. Today, the medical marijuana movement is steadily gathering steam, even as lawmakers fear for their own reelection if they support it. Since 1996, voters in Alaska, Arizona, California, Colorado, Maine, Nevada, Oregon, and Washington have voted in favor of the legalization of cannabis for medical use. Voters in Colorado and Nevada passed ballot initiatives exempting patients from state criminal penalties when they use marijuana under the supervision of a physician. And in the lush, tropical state of Hawaii, the legislature legalized the medical use of marijuana.

The dam holding back the flow of cannabis is leaking from a thousand cracks. Canada has approved legislation that makes it legal to possess and cultivate marijuana for medical purposes for those suffering from terminal illnesses and severe chronic conditions. Under the new rules, people still have to apply for exemptions from the general ban, but the regulations eliminate what used to be standardized limits on how much marijuana someone using it for medical purposes could possess. These limits are now superseded by the recommendations of an individual's personal physician who in effect is authorized to write a prescription for marijuana.

A 1999 Gallup poll showed that 73 percent of all Americans support the medical use of marijuana. A number of medical organizations, including the AIDS Action Council, American Public Health Association, and the state nursing associations of Alaska, California, Colorado, Florida, New Mexico, New York, North Carolina, and Virginia, support prescriptive access to medical marijuana. Cannabis is a medicine—and a good one.

If it is perceived that the Public Health Service is going around and giving marijuana to folks, there would be a perception that this stuff can't be so bad. It gives a bad signal.
—James Mason, M.D., former head of the U.S. Public Health Service

In traditional modalities of medicine such as India's Ayurveda, cannabis has enjoyed millennia of use as a valuable medicine. It is recommended for relief of pain and headaches, for increasing appetite, for promoting sleep in cases of insomnia, for subduing hysteria, and for easing painful menstruation. Until 1941, marijuana was listed in the *U.S. Pharmacopoeia* as an approved drug. Today it's listed as a Schedule I drug, on par with crack and heroin. But the conversation about medical marijuana is intensifying. Research focuses primarily on the efficacy of cannabis in analgesia, relieving nausea and vomiting, counteracting wasting syndrome by means of appetite stimulation, and inhibiting the progress of glaucoma. In each of these areas, cannabis demonstrates real and significant value.

Medical cannabis has many intelligent champions. Clearly the leader of them all is Lester Grinspoon, M.D., a professor of psychiatry at Harvard University whose tireless efforts on behalf of medical marijuana have pushed the conversation very far down the road. His courage, intellectual and scientific rigor, and impeccable credentials have made him a force to reckon with. Dr. Grinspoon says, "The greatest harm in recreational use of marijuana came not from the drug itself but from the effects of prohibition." In hindsight, Dr. Grinspoon says, "I thought clinical research on marijuana would be eagerly pursued. A quarter of a century later, I have begun to doubt this." He and coauthor James Bakalar produced their book *Marihuana: The Forbidden Medicine*, a brilliant reference on the subject that, unlike the WHO report described previously, cannot be suppressed.

Ongoing research brought to light by Dr. Grinspoon and Bakalar and numerous others shows the following beneficial applications of medical cannabis:

Analgesia—Pain is one of the most common conditions for which drug treatment is sought. Pain comes in varied forms. Neuropathic pain is caused by damage or abnormality anywhere along a nerve. Nociceptive pain originates as a result of inflammation around an injury. These two pain types can occur at the same time, depending on the nature of physical damage. Postsurgical pain is very common, affecting almost everybody who undergoes any kind of surgical procedure. Cancer pain is caused by tumor growth into sensitive areas and by cancer surgery and radiation. Whatever the cause, pain can range from mild to completely debilitating. Any agent that can help is valuable.

In almost all painful maladies I have found Indian Hemp by far the most useful of drugs.

—Dr. J. Russell Reynolds, physician to Queen Victoria

Cannabis is an excellent, time-tested analgesic, first brought to light to Westerners by Dr. W. B. O'Shaughnessy in the 1840s. O'Shaughnessy studied the uses of cannabis for pain in Indian traditional medicine and conducted both animal and human experiments for this purpose. In the 19th century, tincture of cannabis was commonly used as an analgesic. Since the mid-1800s, hundreds of articles on the analgesic uses of cannabis have appeared in British and American medical journals. Entities such as the Oakland Cannabis Buyer's Cooperative and the San Francisco Cannabis Buyer's Club dispense medical marijuana to numerous people in need, including for pain relief.

Glaucoma—The most common cause of blindness in the Western world, glaucoma is characterized by increased intraocular pressure. This pressure is caused by a blockage in the channels that regulate the eye's internal fluid. An even balance of fluid maintains the healthy spherical shape of the eye. But increased fluid and pressure can damage the optic nerve, resulting in blindness. In both animals and humans, smoking or eating cannabis results in reduced intraocular pressure. A few studies, and numerous anecdotal reports, indicate that cannabis can play a valuable role in stemming the progress of glaucoma.

Nausea and Wasting Syndrome—There's nothing like a toxic dose of chemotherapy to put you on your knees, clutching the rim of the toilet, head in the bowl, puking your guts out. Chemotherapy makes all your hair fall out, causes tremendous nausea and vomiting, kills appetite, causes serious wasting, and even puts some people in the grave. Plus, it costs a fortune. And it's legal. Cannabis makes people feel good, does none of the above, and kills nobody. It's illegal, and you can be thrown in prison for its use. Go figure.

As far as mitigating nausea and stemming vomiting caused by chemotherapy is concerned, the jury is back on cannabis. In whole cannabis form or as nabilone, the cannabinoids have been shown in several dozen studies to reduce nausea and vomiting in patients suffering from chemotherapy poisoning. The cannabinoids perform as well as or better than other prescription drugs for the same purpose. Without surprise, some studies show that smoked cannabis works better than orally ingested THC pills. If you're nauseous, you're not going to be able to keep a pill down, plus this route of ingestion produces quicker results and a superior nausea-quelling effect. There is no question whatsoever that cannabis reduces vomiting in chemotherapy sufferers.

Another effect of chemotherapy, and a typical effect of AIDS, is wasting due to loss of appetite. For this condition, cannabis is a tremendous boon, promoting appetite in individuals who otherwise have no desire to eat. In studies of chemotherapy sufferers, cannabis improved appetite. Countless AIDS patients have used cannabis for the same purpose, with good results. What compassionate human being on Earth would deny cannabis to these people?

Overall, successful reports from the field far exceed in volume the results yielded by the limited number of clinical tests. Though some people accept only double-blind, placebo-controlled, crossover clinical trials, others accept real-life human experience as valid for sorting out what works and what doesn't—and what cannabis is reported to work on includes menstrual cramps, hypertension, anxiety, muscle spasms, epilepsy, asthma, rheumatic pain, and anxiety. Medicine may not be the primary use of cannabis worldwide, but for those who turn to it for relief from a variety of health disorders, it has been good medicine indeed.

Praise the Lord and Pass the Joint

In October 2000, self-professed pot grower and outspoken cannabis proponent Jonathan Adler invited the governor of Hawaii and local law enforcement officials to attend the opening of the Hawaii Medical Marijuana Institute, a 10,000-square-foot facility dedicated to growing and providing legal cannabis to those with medical needs. Not unexpectedly, Governor Benjamin Caitano didn't show. But Adler garnered some public attention nonetheless, and that was part of the point.

The Puna district of the big island of Hawaii is a major

cannabis growing area. Since 1996, Adler, who lives in Puna, has behaved in exactly the opposite manner of other cannabis growers and dealers. While other growers hide their activities, John Adler has gone to the police, drug enforcement agencies, and government offices to declare that he is a grower and seller. He advertises in the newspaper and has appeared on a number of television programs to state for the record his cannabis-related activities. He grows superpotent pot, and he is proud of that fact.

In 1998, Adler was busted for possession of cannabis. Yet, as of summer 2001 he was still awaiting trial. Local authorities have done everything possible to obfuscate, foot-drag, and delay the court date. For if Adler is tried by a jury of his peers, with his convincing religious and medical views on full display in a region in which cannabis is the number-one cash crop, he will win. Thus, the problem. To the authorities, John Adler is a royal pain in the butt.

Sitting in his living room, John rolls a huge joint of Hawaiian superweed from his own special stock while he describes Hawaii's cannabis dilemma. "Everybody suffers from a condition known as CDS, or cannabis deficiency syndrome. There's only one medicine that can cure it." He raises the giant joint. "Cannabis is the answer. And even though Hawaiians voted in favor of medical marijuana, there's no provision for making it available to people in need. So that's what I'm doing. I operate the only legal, sanctioned facility for medical cannabis in Hawaii. And if I do say so myself, this is first-rate, high-quality medicine." He fires up the imponderable bomber joint and sucks in a few cubic meters of smoke.

An ordained minister since 1974, the Reverend John Adler comes at legal cannabis from two directions. Given Hawaii's provision allowing medical marijuana use by those who pos-

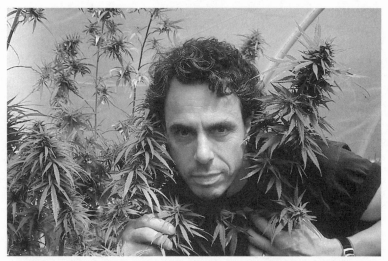

The author goes to pot in John Adler's greenhouse, Puna, Hawaii.

sess the right documentation from a physician, Adler has ap-
pointed himself as a provider, believing that according to the
law, he has a right to do so. But as a backup, he also stands as
the head of a church whose holy sacrament is cannabis. Adler
declares in a church pamphlet: "Our religious liberty dictates
our choices and our mandate insures cannabis use in a spiritual
manner. The law protects free exercise of religion. Amen!"
This same claim is made by the Rastafarians, whose beliefs are
rooted deeply in the Bible and whose politico-religious views
have been well established since the early 1950s.

   Some may dismiss Adler as a crank, but I wouldn't. Bright,
articulate, persuasive, and well-informed, John Adler just may
be the man to pave the way for legal cannabis cultivation and
sales in Hawaii. His form of religious expression is no more
outlandish, and far less dangerous, than fundamentalist snake
handlers or any number of bona fide, albeit fringe, churches.
One thing is certain: We have not heard the last of Reverend
Adler. After drawing heavily on the huge joint, he passes it.
"Worship with me, brother. Praise the Lord."

The Far Horizon

On a hot June morning in Negril, Jamaica, I hopped onto a red Honda motor scooter and weaved my way through the center of town toward the legendary Miss Brown's. I was conducting a survey. I had tried Jenny's special chocolate cannabis cake up on the cliffs near where I was staying. But Miss Brown's was by all accounts the place to go for the most potent space cake on the island. I intended to engage in an argonautic experiment to ascertain the truth for myself. Good science requires personal commitment, you know.

After successfully navigating through crazy traffic, I found myself inside Miss Brown's gaily decorated wooden store getting a rundown on the various psychoactive offerings on the menu. "You ever have Miss Brown's cake?" asked the young Jamaican guy with whom I spoke. I explained that I hadn't, but I had tried the cake at Jenny's. He turned serious and looked me dead in the eye.

"You listen to me, mistuh. I tell you flat out straight truth, no lies, understand? Nobody, I mean nobody, makes the cake like Miss Brown." It was a statement of ponderous import, as if backed by the mighty elemental forces of all nature.

"Okay," I replied. "Then how about a piece of cake to go?" The young man nodded and gave me a look that suggested I had made a wise choice.

Back on the cliffs, I thought to go lightly by eating only half the piece of cake. Properly prepared, cannabis works remarkably quickly when eaten, and not even a half-hour passed when the first tremulous inklings of psychedelic liftoff tickled my nerves. Seated in a comfortable porch chair, thrilling sensations pulled my spine upright, my eyes opened more widely, and my awareness began to expand rapidly. It was a fast takeoff out onto the vast highways of the mind. I could hear every bird along the cliffs, could smell a thousand scents and plants nearby, and could see the most subtle shadings of colors in the trees, water, buildings, and environment around me. I was soaring.

The skin on my face felt as though fine electrical currents were streaming through the tissue. My nostrils felt like tunnels, and the breath blowing through them seemed like a wind from the deepest depths of antiquity. When I dove into the undulating pearlescent blue water of the ocean, my entire body dissolved like sugar. When I sat in the sun, its fire burned in my bones and crackled along every nerve. When I sipped some fine Jamaican Blue Mountain coffee, the smell and taste of all the lush, green vegetation and fruit trees and creeping vines and giant-leafed exotic plants and soft, loamy, rich soil filled my mouth and nose. I was no longer in charge. The gods were taking me on a journey to the far horizon of consciousness, and my part was to take delight in the ride.

Maximizing Cannabis Potency

In 1970, the United States government cannabis program head, Dr. Norman Doorenbos of the University of Mississippi, and his team made a potent discovery. When cannabis is heated to 212°F for 90 minutes, the carboxyl radical is broken off tetrahydrocannabinolic acid, producing THC, and the pot becomes far more potent. Nifty trick. What this means is that you can transform moderately potent ganja into appreciably more potent material by cooking it properly.

This scientific discovery explains why hashish has been steamed in some cultures, and why the heating of cannabis is a fundamental aspect of the preparation of many cannabis electuaries and baked goods. For when cannabis is cooked into cookies and other products, it is rendered more potent.

Ultimate Cannabis Cookies

While cannabis acts most quickly upon the body and mind when smoked, it acts most profoundly when it is eaten. For this reason, writers and poets throughout the ages have waxed effusive on the astonishing ecstasies of eating cannabis as well as its concentrated form, hashish.

To experience for yourself what all the fuss is about, try this recipe for the very finest cannabis cookies in the world. These cookies are not only sensationally delicious and nutritious, but they infuse the mind and body with the reveries of Siva's benefic vibrations.

> 1 stick of butter
> ¼–½ ounce finely ground cannabis (I highly recommend powdering the cannabis in a coffee grinder)
> ½ cup pure maple syrup
> 1 cup almonds, ground in a blender into coarse flour
> ⅓ cup oatmeal, ground in a blender into coarse flour
> ⅓ cup shredded, dried coconut
> ⅓ cup wheat germ
> 1 cup pastry flour
> ¼ teaspoon powdered cinnamon
> Pinch of salt

Place the butter in a pan and melt at low heat. When the butter is thoroughly melted, stir in the finely ground cannabis and simmer it in the butter at low heat for 10 to 15 minutes.

This oil-simmering process is probably the single most important part of preparation. Remove the cannabis butter from the stove, and add the maple syrup to it. Stir thoroughly. Combine all other ingredients in a separate bowl. Then mix the butter-cannabis-syrup mixture into the dry ingredients with a spoon.

When ingredients are thoroughly mixed, fashion between 24 and 36 dome-shaped cookies, and lay them out on a greased cookie sheet. Bake at 350°F for 10 to 12 minutes, until golden brown. Cool and serve.

Caution: These cookies taste extremely delicious, but remember that they are pot cookies. It's always best to start with less, as you can consume more if you choose. Do not make the mistake of eating a whole bunch at once, as you will be truly hammered and begging for divine relief. You should feel the effects within 45 minutes, but wait at least an hour-and-a-half before making the decision to consume more. Don't munch on them like chips. Eat one, or maybe just half of one.

Enjoy these with your friends but *be careful*. Pace yourself. Don't drive. Do listen to music. *Keep these cookies out of the reach of children!* Don't ever secretly dose somebody. Chew thoroughly. Think happy thoughts. Plot and scheme world peace. Wash the dog. Do *not* mow the lawn. Make a day of the experience. Sing silly songs. Finger paint. Play erotic-word Scrabble. Run through the sprinkler.

Dutch Flowers

In Amsterdam, more than 350 coffeeshops operate under guidelines of legal tolerance. In those coffeeshops, you can legally purchase and consume cannabis and hash. And it's no big deal. For the most part, these are small neighborhood

shops where people go to have a smoke and drink a cappuccino. It is a civilized and restrained scene. There is relatively
little crime on the street and virtually none associated with
cannabis.

On a gray January afternoon in Amsterdam, I sat with my
friend Lord Nelson by the large plate-glass window of Dutch
Flowers, a small neighborhood coffeeshop just down the canal
from Hotel Estheria, where we were lodged. Techno trance
music played at moderate volume on a pair of speakers. A cappuccino maker hissed steam at the bar. An attractive young
woman in tight jeans weighed out a couple of grams of skunk
cannabis for two patrons.

*Among these sweets is a kind of electuary made with the
fatty extract [of hashish], figs, dates, and honey. Another very
popular kind, madjoun, has cloves, cinnamon, pepper, musk,
and other similar substances. It is said to be highly stimulating.*

　　　　　　　　—Baron Ernst von Bibra, 19th-century botanist

We sat drinking coffees and sharing a joint of Zenith, one
of many local specialty cannabis hybrids cultivated in the
Netherlands. The smoke was light and fragrant and refreshing, a perfect prelude to a hike across town in the winter
chill over to Hortus Botanicus, the botanical gardens whose
large greenhouses hold a spectacular collection of lush tropical foliage. For half an hour or so, we sat contentedly in the
warmth and good cheer of the coffeeshop, out of a cold wind
blowing off the North Sea.

In Amsterdam, you get a good sense of what things are like when all the hype, hysteria, demonization, and blatant misinformation are stripped away from the conversation about cannabis. For Lord Nelson and myself, the break at Dutch Flowers was a special treat, a pleasurable smoke on a museum-hopping vacation. Cannabis is a friendly plant. It delights the mind and promotes enjoyment. For thousands of years, cannabis has been a happy companion of men and women all over the world, for good reason. Good cannabis promotes a sweet and pleasing reverie.

We drained the last drops of coffee from our cups and stubbed out the Zenith. Lord Nelson nodded with approval. "My compliments to the chef." We both laughed. We donned hats and scarves and gloves and, thus fortified with stimulating caffeine and good smoke, we stepped out the door of the little local coffeeshop and walked away briskly in the bracing cold. We had places to go, and many things to see.

Epilogue
Into the Fire

There is something terribly exhilarating about stepping off perfectly good ground into a burning furnace of uneven volcanic stones made red-hot by tons of blazing timber. As I stood at the edge of the huge fire pit, all my accumulated knowledge of unbendable physical laws and principles dissolved away. My nerves vibrated like struck piano wire. My abdominal muscles quivered. The radiant heat from the fire baked my legs and chest and face. I took two deep breaths, and stepped into the fire. Then—all thoughts, notions, and concepts ceased. There was only fire . . . stone . . . walking.

My close friend Ariipaea Salmon, whom I know as Paea, had walked first. As the *tahua*, the keeper of the fire, he had directed all the preparations leading up to the walk itself, and—most important—he had appealed to the gods and spirits to tame the fire so that we could safely cross the stones. After Paea, Kami walked. A kava grower from the island of Pentecost in the Pacific Islands republic of Vanuatu, Kami was part of the native crew that had prepared the fire, an undertaking of mammoth labor that took a couple weeks. I had hiked remote jungle trails behind Kami at other times, and now I was following him across a fire pit on Vanuatu's capital island of Efate. I had never firewalked before; neither had he. You just never know where you're going to wind up with the people you meet.

Behind me, Jonas and two dozen other men from the Vanuatu villages of Bunlap and Baie Martellie readied themselves to walk. So did Paea's son Heiariki, and Simon Agius, a young man who had worked side by side in the preparations with Paea. Behind all of us, like a sorcerer whose incantations and spells are felt but not seen, lay kava, a plant whose psychoactive potion dissolves the cares of a weary mind and links drinkers with the spirits of ancient gods—and one another.

The history between plants and humans points to a grand closeness. By various means, plants have touched the deepest and most vulnerable parts of the human imagination. They have caused us to perform great feats and labors in their name, carrying and cultivating them all around the world. But the suggestion that the action of plants upon humans is merely physical or chemical strips essential mystic sinew from the corpus of life. Like reading only every other word of a fabulous book, you may catch the drift of the tale, but the full story and its meaning remain unknown. We eat plants, drink their juices, wear their fibers, scent ourselves with their fragrances, build homes and structures with their materials, adorn our property and bodies with them, employ them to alter mind and mood, are attracted by their beauty or oddness, and, sometimes, are deeply moved by them—just as they drew me in to the sacred native ceremonies of the South Pacific and quite literally into the fire.

I never was interested in the firewalking empowerment workshops that became so popular during the New Age. Not that I ever derided the act of firewalking or questioned the danger of doing so. Fire is dangerously hot, whether in a Marin

County backyard or on a remote Pacific island. Call it purist conceit, but I determined that if I ever firewalked, it would be in a traditional native setting. That opportunity arose in the spring of 2000 when Paea called me from Baie Martellie. "Hello, Chris," his resonant voice called through the line. "I have something important to tell you. I have decided to put on a firewalk for the full moon of August. Will you come?" Of course, Paea knew the answer before calling.

Baie Martellie had been heavily damaged in November 1999 by a tsunami generated by a midnight earthquake at sea. Virtually the entire village had been swept away. Baie Martellie is the place where Paea and I first came to know each other. Kava had led me there. I had been investigating *Piper methysticum* for possible extraction and marketing in the United States, and I became friendly with many of the local kava growers, spending many happy hours walking with them in the jungle, preparing and drinking kava, and participating in village life. The natives accepted me wholeheartedly, and I promised to help them over time as I could. When Paea informed me that the firewalk would raise relief funds for Baie Martellie, I had to go and walk.

I booked my passage and wondered what it would be like to step onto red-hot coals. "The fire will be the biggest one ever in Vanuatu," Paea assured me. "I will build a pit at least 15 meters [50 feet] long. The fire will be very powerful, very cleansing."

My first time walking across the 12-foot width of the fire, I burned a spot on the arch of my right foot. But I was not willing to let that be my only firewalking experience. Three subsequent times across the same stones, I walked without mishap. When I lined up with Paea and the Pentecost Island villagers, we walked the full length of the pit. The glowing stones were hot enough to fry a steak. Flames licked up from between the rocks. The uneven footing would have made walking precarious even without a fire. In the roasting heat of the pit, where 40 tons of timber burned beneath 50 tons of volcanic stones, we should have been immolated. Yet, together we walked on safely.

I have heard a few humorous explanations for firewalking. One is that you get into a mental state in which you are impervious to burning. Another is that the incipient sweating of the soles of the feet prevents burning by creating a thin film of moisture on the skin. I have even been told that volcanic stones never really get that hot, or that a fine layer of ash settles upon the stones and prevents burning. All of these wonderfully absurd theories arise, of course, from those who have not walked.

The world is filled with people who engage in direct action and those who speculate, theorize, second-guess, postulate, and concoct myriad abstract notions. Those who are engaged share an advantage that the theoreticians can never get close to; they know what it is like to throw oneself wholeheartedly into an activity. The others do not.

I believe that the simple truth of firewalking so stretches the boundaries of the mind that most people would rather believe in the silly theories above. I accept that the "secret" to firewalking is exactly as natives describe it: You build a huge fire, you acknowledge the gods and spirits, they tame the fire for your passage, and you walk on safely. This spiritual protection saves the firewalker from horrible injury or death.

Herein lies not just the secret to firewalking but to life itself. It is altogether too easy to accept a neat and tidy interpretation of life devoid of all mystery, a linear, logical, practical explanation. But such an explanation does not accommodate love, god, mystic revelation, or any of the most grand and potent experiences in life. What about exploring life's mysteries head-on? We explore outer space, but what about delving into inner space? In the 1960s, millions of us ingested or otherwise consumed psychoactive substances, and we discovered that there are many joyful, ingenious, inspiring dimensions to the human mind that we had not encountered in church or social studies class. This is where the psyche delicacies come in. These plants provide us with the means to safely tinker with our minds, to experience refreshing and delightful states of being, to revel, to play, to enjoy. And here's the big question: If life isn't enjoyable, what the heck are we doing? Throw yourself wholeheartedly into exploration and you just may make some marvelous discoveries. Why not?

Magic works as long as there are those who accept it and commit bold acts by it. And the magic dies out when there are no longer any believers.

Further Reading

Andrews, Jean. *Peppers: The Domesticated Capsicums*. Austin: University of Texas Press, 1995.

Clarke, Robert Connell. *Hashish*. Los Angeles: Red Eye Press, 1998.

Coe, Sophie, and Michael Coe. *The True History of Chocolate*. London: Thames & Hudson, 1996.

Cooke, Mordecai C. *The Seven Sisters of Sleep*. 1860. Lincoln, MA: Quarterman Publications, 1991.

Dulcinos, Donald P. *Pioneer of Inner Space: The Life of Fitz Hugh Ludlow, Hasheesh Eater*. Brooklyn, NY: Autonomedia, 1998.

Grinspoon, Lester, and James Bakalar. *Marihuana: The Forbidden Medicine*. New Haven: Yale University Press, 1997.

Huxley, Aldous. *The Doors of Perception*. New York: Harper & Brothers, 1954.

Jacob, H. E. *Coffee: The Epic of a Commodity*. New York: Viking Press, 1962.

Kilham, Christopher. *Kava: Medicine Hunting in Paradise*. Rochester, VT: Park Street Press, 1996.

Lamb, F. Bruce. *Rio Tigre and Beyond: The Amazon Jungle Medicine of Manuel Cordova*. Berkeley, CA: North Atlantic Books, 1985.

———. *Wizard of the Upper Amazon*. Berkeley, CA: North Atlantic Books, 1987.

Lebot, Vincent, Mark Merlin, and Lamont Lindstrom. *Kava: The Pacific Drug*. New Haven: Yale University Press, 1992.

Lewin, Louis. *Phantastica*. 1924. Rochester, VT: Park Street Press, 1988.

McKenna, Terence. *Food of the Gods*. New York: Bantam Books, 1992.

————. *True Hallucinations.* San Francisco: Harper Odyssey, 1993.

Ott, Jonathan. *Pharmacotheon: Entheogenic Drugs, Their Plant Sources and History.* Kennewick, WA: Natural Products Company, 1993.

Pendergrast, Mark. *Uncommon Grounds: The History of Coffee and How It Transformed Our World.* New York: Basic Books, 1999.

Plotkin, Mark. *Tales of a Shaman's Apprentice.* New York: Penguin Books, 1993.

Schivelbusch, Wolfgang. *Tastes of Paradise.* New York: Vintage Books, 1993.

Schultes, Richard Evans, and Albert Hofmann. *Plants of the Gods.* New York: Alfred van der Marck Editions, 1979.

Sherman, Carol, Andrew Smith, and Erik Tanner. *Highlights: An Illustrated History of Cannabis.* Berkeley, CA: Ten Speed Press, 1999.

Strausbaugh, John, and Donald Blaise, eds. *The Drug User: Documents, 1840–1960.* New York: Blast Books, 1991.

Tedlock, Dennis, trans. *Popol Vuh: The Mayan Book of the Dawn of Life.* New York: Touchstone Books, 1996.

von Bibra, Baron Ernst. *Plant Intoxicants.* 1855. Rochester, VT: Healing Arts Press, 1995.

Weil, Andrew. *The Natural Mind.* New York: Houghton Mifflin, 1973.

————, and Winifred Rosen. *From Chocolate to Morphine.* New York: Houghton Mifflin, 1983.

Index

About the Author

Chris Kilham is the founder of Medicine Hunter, Inc. He conducts research expeditions around the world to discover and develop new medicines, botanical health products, and educational programs for the natural products market and the media. Chris is the author of 12 books and has appeared as a guest on hundreds of radio and television programs. He is an inveterate body surfer, yogi, traveler, and pleasure seeker. He lives in Massachusetts.